# First-Time Parents Box Set

*Becoming a Dad + Newborn Care Basics - Pregnancy Preparation for Dads-to-Be and Expecting Moms*

**Lisa Marshall**

© Copyright 2019 by Lisa Marshall - All rights reserved.

This book is provided with the sole purpose of providing relevant information on a specific topic for which every reasonable effort has been made to ensure that it is both accurate and reasonable. Nevertheless, by purchasing this book you consent to the fact that the author, as well as the publisher, are in no way experts on the topics contained herein, regardless of any claims as such that may be made within. As such, any suggestions or recommendations that are made within are done so purely for entertainment value. It is recommended that you always consult a professional prior to undertaking any of the advice or techniques discussed within.

This is a legally binding declaration that is considered both valid and fair by both the Committee of Publishers Association and the American Bar Association and should be considered as legally binding within the United States.

The reproduction, transmission, and duplication of any of the content found herein, including any specific or extended information will be done as an illegal act regardless of the end form the information ultimately takes. This includes copied versions of the work both physical, digital and audio unless the express consent of the Publisher is provided beforehand. Any additional rights reserved.

Furthermore, the information that can be found within the pages described forthwith shall be considered both accurate and truthful when it comes to the recounting of facts. As such, any use, correct or incorrect, of the provided information will render the Publisher free of responsibility as to the actions taken outside of their direct purview. Regardless, there are zero scenarios where the original author or the Publisher can be deemed liable in any fashion for any damages or hardships that may result from any of the information discussed herein.

Additionally, the information in the following pages is intended only for informational purposes and should thus be thought of as universal. As befitting its nature, it is presented without assurance regarding its prolonged validity or interim quality. Trademarks that are mentioned are done without written consent and can in no way be considered an endorsement from the trademark holder.

**CHAPTER 7: FIRST TRIMESTER — CONCEPTION THROUGH 12 WEEKS** ..... 73

**CHAPTER 8: SECOND TRIMESTER — *13 TO 27 WEEKS*** ............................................. 89

**CHAPTER 9: THIRD TRIMESTER — *28 TO 40 WEEKS*** ............................................. 103

**CHAPTER 10: COMPLICATIONS IN PREGNANCY** ............................................. 122

**CHAPTER 11: GOING INTO LABOR** ...... 144

**CHAPTER 12: WHO'S GOING TO BE THERE WHEN THE BABY COMES?** ...... 152

**CHAPTER 13: CHILDBIRTH METHODS AND GEAR** .............................................. 160

**CHAPTER 14: COMPLICATIONS IN LABOR AND CHILDBIRTH** ..................... 171

**CHAPTER 15: THE BIRTH ITSELF** ........ 184

**CHAPTER 16: CESAREAN SECTION** ..... 204

**CHAPTER 17: COMPLICATIONS AFTER DELIVERY** ............................................. 214

**CHAPTER 18: NOW YOU HAVE A BABY!** ................................................................ 217

**CHAPTER 19: BABY CARE AT HOME** ... 233

**CHAPTER 20: PARENTAL CARE AT HOME** ................................................................ 248

**CONCLUSION** .......................................... 261

# Newborn Care Basics:

*Baby Care Tips For New Moms*

**INTRODUCTION** .................................... 265

**CHAPTER 1: BONDING WITH BABY** .... 268

**CHAPTER 2: FEEDING A NEWBORN** ... 305

**CHAPTER 3: NEWBORN SLEEP** ........... 343

**CHAPTER 4: CLEANING BABY** ............. 376

**CHAPTER 5: CARING FOR NEWBORN BELLY BUTTON** ...................................... 404

**CHAPTER 6: CLOTHING BABY..............417**

**CHAPTER 7: CARING FOR A CIRCUMCISION .....................................443**

**CONCLUSION .......................................459**

# BECOMING A DAD

# The First-Time Dad's Guide to Pregnancy Preparation

## (101 Tips for Expectant Dads)

Author

Lisa Marshall

# DAD

*"A son's first hero, a daughter's first love"*

# Introduction

## *You're having a baby!*

There are two kinds of pregnancies: The planned, and the unplanned.

If you and your partner have been trying to get pregnant—congrats! You're embarking on life's greatest adventure together.

And if you and your partner have been trying *not* to get pregnant—still congrats! You might not have thought you were ready yet, but it's still going to be an adventure.

Planned or unplanned, finding out you have a baby on the way is just the first step on a journey that will take you places you never imagined. But no need to panic! Generations of men before you have become dads and lived to tell the tale. You can do this, too. This book will cover everything you need to know about pregnancy, childbirth and what comes afterward.

The key is to know something about what's going to happen next, so you can get ready. Sure, your partner is doing the heavy lifting physically, but you're in this together and your participation is mission-critical. So strap in, because it's gonna be a bumpy ride. But the payoff is unbelievable.

# Chapter 1:
# How do you know she is pregnant?

Most likely your partner purchased a home pregnancy test. When she opened the box she found a stick that looked something like a digital thermometer. She was instructed to pee on the stick, wait a few minutes, and check the little window. The window might show lines, or negative or positive signs, or even the words "pregnant" or "not pregnant."

This kind of pregnancy test works by checking the urine for a hormone called human chorionic gonadotropin (hCG). When a fertilized egg settles into the uterus, the cells that will become the placenta start making this hormone. The amount of hCG being made doubles every 72 hours up until about 12 weeks into pregnancy. By the time your partner realized her period was late, there was enough hCG in her urine to show up on a home pregnancy test.

## *Are home pregnancy tests always accurate?*

Pregnancy tests are pretty darn accurate, but nothing in life is 100%.

In the early days of home pregnancy tests, a woman had to wait until her period was at least a couple of weeks late. Then, she had to limit how much she drank the night before and test her urine first thing in the morning. That was all to make sure the level of hCG in her urine was high enough for the test.

Now, she can test on the day her period should start (possibly even before) and she can do the test any time of day. This is because the technology for detecting hCG has become extremely sensitive.

However, test results aren't accurate every single time. It isn't common, but there can be both false negatives (she's pregnant, but the test says she isn't) and false positives (she's not pregnant, but the test says she is).

## *What causes a false negative?*

A negative result can be disappointing—or a huge relief. It can also be inaccurate if the woman is pregnant but there's not enough hCG in her urine for the test to pick up on. While today's tests are way more sensitive than they were in the past, they still have limits.

It's important to read the instructions that come with the test. She can get a false negative if she takes the test too soon, if her urine is too diluted or if she just doesn't wait long enough to check the stick for the result.

## *What causes a false positive?*

A positive result can bring joy or sorrow. But again, while they are even less common than false negatives, false positives can occur.

Many pregnancies end early, even before the woman suspects she is pregnant. The fertilized egg may have attached to the uterus but for some reason just didn't take. An early test may pick up on hCG from a pregnancy that has already ended.

Sometimes a fertilized egg attaches someplace outside the uterus, in what's known as an ectopic pregnancy. Ectopic pregnancies can go away on their own, but often they have to be removed surgically because they can be life-threatening for the woman.

Some medications can cause false-positive results. This obviously includes hormone treatments, but it also includes a few that might surprise you, like methadone and some antidepressants.

Some medical conditions can lead to false positives, especially if they cause white or red blood cells to show up in the urine.

*How do you confirm a home pregnancy test result?*

If the result is positive, or if it's negative but your partner still thinks she might be pregnant, she can always wait a week or two and take another test. Many tests come in packages of two for just this reason.

However, if she's having worrisome symptoms like pain or unusual bleeding, or if it's important to know about a pregnancy as soon as possible, she can see a healthcare provider for confirmation. She can see her regular primary care provider or go to a Planned Parenthood clinic. She should be cautious about going to a "crisis pregnancy center" as these places often provide inaccurate or incomplete information.

Most healthcare providers test urine using the very same technology as home pregnancy tests. They don't usually do blood tests for pregnancy, but they may do them for other reasons.

Depending on how far along the pregnancy is thought to be, a physical exam may be done. They may have your partner lay down on an examining table, then press on her belly to see if her uterus is enlarged. They may do an internal exam to look at her cervix, the lower part of her uterus. In pregnancy, the cervix will soften and change color.

If the pregnancy is far enough along, they may check for a heartbeat. After about 10 weeks it may be possible to pick up the baby's heartbeat with a handheld device called a Doppler, which is kind of like an audio-only ultrasound. Some midwives like to go old school with a Pinard horn, an ancient kind of stethoscope that looks something like a really skinny Pilsner glass.

And of course, for the ultimate audio-visual experience, they may do an ultrasound. Early on, six to eight weeks or so, ultrasounds are usually done trans-vaginally, with a slender device inserted into the vagina. Not every woman is going to be okay with that, and it isn't usually done unless there's an important reason for it.

Otherwise, she is likely to be offered a trans-abdominal ultrasound at around 12 weeks. This is the less-intrusive kind they show on TV, where the device is passed over her belly. At this early stage, you'll definitely hear a heartbeat but the visuals may be hard to figure out. Sometimes you see something that really looks like a baby, but sometimes it's a lot of static and you have to take the technician's word for it!

The ultimate in ultrasound tech is the 3D format. It produces a picture that's so eerily lifelike it almost feels voyeuristic like you should give the little guy some privacy. (But instead, it'll probably go straight to Instagram.)

## *What are the symptoms of early pregnancy?*

Long before she starts looking pregnant, your partner will start feeling the effects of the flow of pregnancy hormones. Typical symptoms include:

- Nausea, sometimes with vomiting
- Feeling bloated and gassy
- Very tender breasts

- Fatigue
- Sensitivity to smells and tastes that didn't bother her before
- Headaches
- Feeling emotional

This may not sound like much fun, and for many women, it really isn't much fun. Fortunately, she should start feeling better within a few weeks.

Typically, pregnancy lasts about nine calendar months, and it's divided into three parts, called trimesters. An old saying, "Three months dreary, three months cheery and three months weary," describes it pretty well.

During those first three months—the first trimester—your partner may feel tired, cranky and weepy. In the second trimester the earlier discomforts usually start to resolve, and she may start to really enjoy being pregnant. Her energy comes back, she enjoys food again and she has a proud little baby bump. In the last trimester, she may start having new discomforts owing to the size of the baby and its weight as it presses on her bladder and diaphragm, and she might start counting the days until the baby comes and she has her body back.

More about all of this soon.

## *What if the pregnancy fails?*

When a pregnancy ends unexpectedly before 20 weeks, this is known as a miscarriage. About 10 percent to 20 percent of known pregnancies end in miscarriage, usually in the first trimester. After 12 weeks the risk of miscarriage decreases dramatically. This is why many couples will wait until 12 weeks to start telling friends and family that they're expecting.

It's estimated that about 50 percent to 75 percent of pregnancies actually end before the woman even knows she's pregnant. When this happens, her period is usually on time or perhaps a little late. She may or may not have more cramping than usual.

Having a miscarriage after the pregnancy has been confirmed can cause emotions from sadness to devastation, depending on how much it was wanted. Even if the pregnancy was unintended and neither of you were really happy about it, you might find an early miscarriage leaves you with a surprising mixture of relief and sadness.

If you've told others that you were expecting, you may dread having to now tell them there's not going to be a baby after all. This can be hard to do, but may also bring some comfort. It is very likely that many women you know have had miscarriages they never talked about; they'll talk about them now, and you'll realize how common this experience really is.

# Chapter 2: Getting ready to be parents

When you were a kid, *parents* were old people of an earlier generation. They were adults and they did adult stuff, like going to work, and mowing the lawn, and never running out of toilet paper.

It might be impossible to imagine your parents as a young couple, living wild and free. But what you are now, they once were—and what they are now, you will be.

Impossible, right? Yeah, that's what your dad thought, too, when he was in your shoes.

You're going to be a dad. And your partner is going to be a mom—if you feel intimidated, imagine how she feels! Fortunately, you're a team. You're going to figure this out together.

First, though, to be the best parents you can be you need to make sure you take care of yourselves and each other. Before getting into the details of parenthood, let's talk about how to protect and strengthen your relationship.

## *Taking a babymoon*

### *What's a babymoon?*

If you're married, you may or may not have had a honeymoon—time away, just the two of you, to revel in your new status. Back in the day, getting married meant spending nights alone together for the first time. A honeymoon was important for figuring out how to be a couple.

Nowadays most couples have spent nights together before the wedding; in fact, they have likely lived together. A honeymoon is still nice, though, because being married is still a change from not being married.

A babymoon is based on the same kind of idea. However long you've been together, becoming parents means a dramatic change in your relationship. What you're gaining will far outweigh what you're losing, but one part of your life is ending forever: the part where it's just the two of you. A babymoon is a celebration of both the life you're leaving behind and the life you're about to begin.

*How long should a babymoon be?*

This is entirely up to you. If you want to take your dream trip together, go for it. If you are limited by time and money, keep it simple. Some couples will check off an exotic bucket-list destination, and some will spend a quiet weekend not too far from home. The point is to be together, knowing that big changes are coming.

*When should you take your babymoon?*

Again, this is up to you. Besides practicalities of time and money, consider the physical demands of pregnancy. If you want to go on a long journey, engage in strenuous activities or go where medical care is not readily available, you'll probably want to aim for the second trimester, between 12 and 20 weeks. That way you'll be past the discomforts of early pregnancy and highest risk of miscarriage, and not yet into the discomforts of late pregnancy or chance of early labor.

If you're going for a quiet weekend close to home and you want to have your babymoon nearer to the baby's arrival, you can wait until the last trimester. At that point, you'll be very aware of the huge leap you're about to take together, and this time together can feel especially meaningful.

## *Sex*

Do you both love spontaneous romantic gestures? Still savor wild, passionate nights and long, lazy mornings in bed? Have just a few spots left in the house where you haven't enjoyed an unplanned quickie?

No one's saying you can't have any of that after the baby comes. It's just that you probably won't—not for a while, at least. It's okay, that's normal.

But what about sex while your partner is pregnant?

## *Is it okay to have sex during pregnancy?*

In rare cases, there may be complications with a pregnancy that puts sex off-limits, at least for some period of time. But for the most part, sex is perfectly safe for the baby, even late into the third trimester. If babies in the uterus could not survive the normal activities of mom's daily life, humans would have died out long ago.

Generally speaking, the only thing limiting your sexual activity is how sexy you and your partner feel. This is likely to change throughout the pregnancy, and you may not always be in sync. Sometimes you'll be turned on by her growing breasts, but they'll be so sore she can't stand for you to touch them. Sometimes her surging hormones will make her super horny, but feeling the baby move as she pulls you closer makes you go limp.

As with every aspect of your relationship, honesty (and a sense of humor) is critical. Talk to each other, take it day by day, and don't compare yourself to what others say they're doing.

# Chapter 3:
# Talking about the future

Maybe you were one of those couples who found out on the first date that your parenting philosophies were in perfect sync. Maybe you both came from loving, healthy families. Maybe your own parents were such excellent role models you know exactly how it all works.

Or maybe when you first starting dating neither of you had ever imagined having kids of your own. Maybe your own parents weren't such great role models, and most of what you learned from them was what *not* to do. Maybe now that a baby is on the way, you're beginning to suspect you're not on the same page at all.

Life doesn't always proceed according to plan, and not all the decisions you make are going to pan out. There will be unforeseen twists and turns, and from time to time you'll need to rethink how you thought things would go.

Your feelings, and your partner's feelings, about many aspects of parenting, will change with time and experience. The key to parenting, as with so many other things in life, is to have a plan—while remaining flexible.

## *Some things to consider—for now*

*Will one (or both) of you stay home?*
Do you have the luxury of allowing one of you to stay home full-time with the baby? If so,

who will it be? Will you take turns? Keep in mind that caring for an infant is a full-time job in itself. Trying to work from home while being solely responsible for the baby's care can be far more difficult than you might imagine. At least, in the beginning, plan to keep baby care and work separately.

If either or both of you have jobs that offer paid parental leave, take it! In some fields, it might mean your career trajectory takes a hit, but this is changing. And you know it's true that no one ever lays on their death bed wishing they'd spent more time at the office. Getting paid to stay home with your new family is a given in some cultures, but in others, it's a rare gift to be treasured.

## *Will you use daycare?*

At some point, you may both need to return to work. Can you arrange your schedules so one of you is always with the baby? This may seem like the ideal arrangement, but if either or both of you work outside the home, it may mean you never see each other during waking hours. That can take a serious toll on your relationship.

The alternative is to have someone else look after the baby while you both work. Unless you have family willing and able to do this, it means hiring someone. Will you get a nanny or au pair who comes to your home? Will you drop the baby off at daycare? Will it be licensed daycare in someone else's home, or at a commercial daycare center? Do either of your workplaces offer childcare?

Of course, while considering your options you'll need to take into account how much childcare will cost. Full-time daycare can be shockingly expensive! You may find it's actually more affordable for one of you to stay home, at least for a while. In any case, it's important to discuss these topics openly and be on the same page.

## *How will household duties be shared?*

Ever see one of those old TV shows where the husband complains he works hard all day while the wife gets to stay home and chill, while the wife complains the husband gets to kick back in the office all day while she works her fingers to the bone? Then they swap places, and neither can handle what the other does?

Reality is, of course, somewhere in the middle. Maybe you can't wait to go to work each day, and you come home feeling refreshed and energetic. Or maybe you come home feeling exhausted and brain-dead, craving a cold beer and some mindless TV. Either way, you might feel you've done enough for the day and deserve some time off.

But if you've ever been the partner at home with the baby all day, you know full-on parenting is at least as exhausting as working outside the home. When your partner walks in the door at the end of the day you may be ready to hand over that baby and head for the hills.

And yet, stuff still needs to be done. Cooking, dishes, laundry, oil changes . . . unless you are lucky enough to have hired help, it's up to the two of you. The time to figure out who's going to do what is now, not when you find yourself in crisis.

## *Some things to consider—for later*

As your child grows, there will be more decisions to be made. You don't have to settle these right now but start the conversation now to avoid surprises later.

### *What's your philosophy on discipline?*

This is likely to be based on your own upbringing, whether you want to follow your parents' example or defy it, and the same will be true for your partner.

Some children are so naturally well-behaved they need little in the way of guidance, but what if yours is a hellion? How will you handle defiance and misbehavior? Do you believe in spanking? Time-outs? Withholding allowance or favorite activities? Can you control your own temper when dealing with a misbehaving child?

## *What kind of schooling do you want your child to have?*

There are so many choices! Public school, private school, parochial school, homeschooling, unschooling, online schooling . . . Where your child ends up will to some degree depend on his or her personality, interests and abilities, but you and your partner are bound to have some strong feelings about how you want your child educated.

## *How will you approach gender expectations?*

When you were a kid, gender differences were probably pretty well defined. Even with a liberal upbringing, boys were boys and girls were girls. Clothing stores, toy aisles and recess activities were clearly segregated. There were two genders, and everyone identified as one or the other.

Whether you find it liberating or distressing, gender roles and expectations—even the very definition of gender—are changing. At the same time, Instagram is overflowing with expectant parents outdoing each other in the scale of their gender-reveal parties. People are still going to ask you if you're having a boy or a girl.

Do you want to find out the sex of your baby before its born? Are you going to buy clothing and decorations that are pink and frilly, or blue and bold? Or are you going to decorate and buy newborn outfits in neutral yellows and greens and be surprised when the baby comes?

And once you know, what then? Are you going to encourage your daughter to take ballet, or your son to play football? Are you going to leave all options on the table and let them decide? What if they don't know if they want to be a boy or a girl? Or they identify as something that doesn't match their genitals? What if your child is intersex, and not clearly either male or female?

Of course, you won't have answers to all these questions immediately. Some will be easier to answer when you know your child better, and some will, in time, answer themselves. What's important now is to talk about how you'll approach these sensitive issues, and how you'll support your child regardless of gender.

## *What about healthcare matters?*

This used to be a no-brainer. Boys were circumcised, or not, depending largely on the family tradition. Everyone followed the recommended vaccination schedule, and everyone who had access to regular dental care got routine X-rays, fillings and fluoride treatments.

Nowadays, though, parents are less likely to accept conventional wisdom without asking questions. You and your partner will want to make well-informed decisions about your child's health, but it will be challenging to know if you're getting reliable information. Now is the time to see where you both stand on healthcare matters, and to agree on trusted sources you'll turn to when you need to know more.

# Chapter 4:
# Early preparations

## *Diet*

Is a pregnant woman "eating for two?" Kind of . . . but not really.

In the first trimester, a woman doesn't usually need to take in any extra calories. The baby-to-be is just an embryo at this stage and doesn't need a lot in the way of building materials. If she has morning sickness or is having trouble handling the way things taste, she should eat what she can.

In the second and third trimesters, she needs to take in about 400 to 500 extra calories per day. Those extra calories can come from larger portions of her regular meals, or from healthy between-meal snacks. Many women find several small meals each day to sit better with them than a few large ones, especially as the baby grows and begins pressing on her internal organs.

A woman can follow any kind of diet that provides the nutrients she and the baby need. "Diet" means vegan, vegetarian, flexitarian, omnivore, etc. It definitely does not mean weight-loss! If your partner is overweight when she gets pregnant she may be advised to limit how much she gains, but this is not the time to try to lose weight.

## *Prenatal vitamins*

Most women will take a prenatal vitamin while pregnant. If the pregnancy was planned, she may have started taking vitamins while trying to conceive. She may well continue taking them after the baby is born, too, especially if she breastfeeds.

Prenatal vitamins contain all the nutrients found in regular multivitamins plus some that are especially important in pregnancy. Most prenatal vitamins have iron, for example, to help keep mom from becoming anemic. Anemia, or not enough red blood cells, is common in pregnancy because so many more are needed to make sure the baby is getting its share. Another critical nutrient is folic acid, which helps prevent birth defects in the baby's brain and spine.

## *Alcohol*

The advice women have been given over the years about drinking during pregnancy has varied. We know that when a pregnant woman drinks, some alcohol reaches the baby. We know alcohol can contribute to miscarriage, stillbirth and health problems in the baby. What we don't know is how much alcohol it takes to cause these problems.

The current medical consensus is that there is no amount of alcohol that is known to be safe during pregnancy, nor any stage of pregnancy when it's known to be safe to drink. Therefore, women who are pregnant, or trying to become pregnant, are advised to avoid alcohol altogether.

Obviously, this isn't a problem if your partner doesn't drink anyway. If she does drink regularly— especially if she has trouble limiting how much she drinks—this will present a special challenge.

Heavy drinking during pregnancy can cause severe, life-long disability in your child. These disabilities are now known as fetal alcohol spectrum disorders (FASDs) and include problems with vision and hearing, low IQ, learning disabilities, ADHD and problems with the heart and kidneys, among many others.

If your partner drinks, make sure she understands the risks this presents. Trying to police and control her behavior is unlikely to be successful, and may just strain your relationship. Suggest she talks to her doctor, midwife or another healthcare provider about getting help. Perhaps she'll be willing to try AA.

You can help make this easier for her by also giving up alcohol until the baby comes. Look for non-alcoholic alternatives to the drinks you both enjoy, and be sure to bring them along to social gatherings where alcohol will be served.

## *Mercury*

Not all forms of mercury are equally toxic. The kind that becomes an issue in pregnancy is called methylmercury, which can cross the placenta and cause serious injury to the developing baby. Methylmercury finds its way into the ocean both through natural processes and through human activity. This most dangerous form of mercury can accumulate in large predatory fish like sharks, swordfish and king mackerel, and pregnant women should avoid eating these. Other kinds of seafood like shrimp, salmon and albacore tuna are less likely to contain dangerous amounts of methylmercury and may be eaten in moderation. Of course, there's no problem here if your partner doesn't care for seafood anyway.

## *Exercise*

Regular exercise is important during pregnancy, both to maintain mental and physical fitness and to prepare for childbirth. If your partner was very active before she got pregnant she will probably want to stay active now. If she didn't get much exercise before it may be a challenge, but all three of you will be better off if she gets up and moving. If she ends up on bedrest or has physical disabilities that limit her mobility, she'll need some expert advise on how to stay fit.

Early pregnancy often brings nausea (and sometimes vomiting) and fatigue. Your partner may also find her stamina lagging and have trouble with activities that demand cardiovascular fitness, like cycling, running and cross-country skiing. This can be frustrating for both of you, but you can usually look forward to the return of her normal energy level once she's out of the first trimester. In late pregnancy, of course, she may have to cut back on some activities as the size of her belly and the change in her center of gravity require some adjustments.

Swimming can be a great form of exercise that easily accommodates her changing body. Depending on where you live there may be yoga, pilates and other exercise classes specifically designed for pregnant women. The ultimate form of exercise for the pregnant woman though (assuming her mobility is not otherwise limited), is walking.

Walking can be relaxing or invigorating—or both! It's good for the heart, lungs, bones, and muscles and can clear her head and lift her mood. It's especially beneficial to the muscles she'll be using during childbirth; in fact, she will likely be encouraged to keep walking while she's in labor. You can do your part by going with her or, if she's really craving some time to herself, helping clear her schedule so she can get out on her own.

## *Are there any kinds of exercise she can't do?*

You're likely to hear a lot of advice and opinions on what kinds of physical activity a pregnant woman should or shouldn't engage in. This is very individual, and commonsense, fitness level and previous experience will be determining factors. Pregnancy is probably not the time to take up water skiing or horseback riding, for example, but if these are activities she loves and does well, she probably won't want to give them up. Some women run marathons—and even triathlons—while pregnant!

Of course, unexpected complications can end up limiting how much she can do, and even the most fit woman is likely to reach a point where the physical demands of pregnancy force her to slow down a bit.

# Chapter 5:
# Finances

Nothing brings financial matters into focus like impending parenthood. Whether by nature you're a spender or a saver, a planner or a freewheeler, decisions must be made. As with everything involved in getting ready for your first child, the key is to have a plan while remaining flexible—because nothing ever goes according to plan.

Money is the number one source of conflict between partners of all kinds, and fighting over finances can be a relationship killer. Talk about this stuff now, make a plan, and get on the same page. It's important for all three of you.

## *Parental leave*

(This is for informational purposes only and is not legal or career advice. Check your employer's policies and your state's laws to determine what kind of leave you are entitled to.)

Many countries understand that society benefits from helping families off to a healthy start, but unfortunately, the US is not one of them. The Family and Medical Leave Act (FMLA) of 1993 is a federal law that requires most, but not all, employers to allow both men and women 12 weeks of parental leave per year. Your employer-provided health insurance has to continue during that time as well. Sounds pretty good, right?

The first problem is that this only means they have to let you come back to work, either to the same position or an equivalent one, after 12 weeks. What they don't have to do is pay you for any part of that 12 weeks.

The second problem is that this only applies to some employers, and to some employees. All public employers, including schools, have to allow parental leave. But private employers only have to comply if they have at least 50 employees.

Then, if your employer is subject to FMLA, the question is do *you* qualify for parental leave. The answer is yes only if you've worked for the employer for at least 12 months (they don't have to be 12 months in a row) and have worked for at least 1,250 hours in the 12 months before your leave starts. Additionally, there must be at least 50 other employees working within 75 miles of where you work.

Keep in mind FMLA is federal law and applies to the bare minimum of what you are entitled to, regardless of where in the US you live. However, you or your employer may be subject to additional state laws, union contracts and other industry-specific requirements. Depending on where you live and what field you work in, you may be entitled to some amount of paid parental leave.

Of course, your employer is free to grant you parental leave if they want to. They can even pay you—if they want to. Some companies do offer paid parental leave as a perk. If your or your partner's employer doesn't, you can always try to negotiate some.

If your job includes paid vacation and sick leave, another option is to try to save it all up and use it during your leave. If you want to use paid time off to extend your leave beyond 12 weeks you can ask, but your employer doesn't have to agree to it. In some states, employers can require you to apply your accrued paid time off to your parental leave.

## *Stretching your parental leave dollar*

### *Stocking up*

You may be the exception, but most of us are better at spending money than saving it. This is one time when you can use this to your advantage, though. Rather than trying to put aside money for all the food and other supplies you'll need while one or both of you are on leave, think about what you'll need and buy as much as you can ahead of time. Fill up your garage and closets with all the non-perishable food, paper goods, toiletries, cleaning supplies and baby stuff you're going to need. You may still be broke at the end, but at least you'll have toilet paper.

*Equal pay plans and paying ahead*

Do you have heating bills that spike in winter, or cooling bills that explode in summer? Talk to your utility companies about getting on equal payment plans. They will average out your annual costs and break them down into 12 equal payments. Sure, that means you don't get those nice shoulder season months where gas and electric are close to nil, but it's much easier to budget for bills that are the same every month.

Whether you go with an equal payment plan or not, you can pay ahead on utility bills. Calculate how much each will be while you and/or your partner are on leave, and add that amount in when you pay your regular bill. You can do that all at once or pay a little extra each month.

## *Rainy day funds*

You've heard that life is what happens while you're busy making other plans. In spite of all your hard work getting ready for this baby, you may find yourself facing expenses you didn't anticipate. It can be difficult, if not impossible, to put money aside when there are already so many financial demands on you.

Brainstorm with your partner and come up with a plan for dealing with financial emergencies. If you can't stuff your mattress with cash, maybe you can have a credit card tucked away that you don't normally use. If you're homeowners, see if you can set up a line of credit on your house.

## *Education savings account*

It's never too soon to start saving up for your child's education. In fact, through the magic of compound interest, even small amounts paid into a modest interest-bearing savings account will add up substantially over 18 years or so. You have other options, though.

Currently, there are two kinds of educational savings accounts, known as Coverdell Education Savings Accounts (ESAs) and 529 plans. They are different from each other in how you invest your money, and they have different rules on matters such as your income level.

This kind of accounts generally earns a better return on investment than an old school savings account. Even better, as long as you only withdraw the principal and earnings for approved educational purposes, you'll never pay taxes on it. As with a 401(k), the money is still yours and you can still withdraw it for other purposes, but you'll pay penalties.

The laws on this kind of accounts change from time to time, so you'll need to research current regulations. You might consider talking to an investment or financial counselor.

## *Life insurance*

The impending arrival of a new life may not seem like the most likely time to think about death. Part of approaching parenthood as responsible adults, though, is thinking about—and planning for—the unthinkable. It's stressful enough figuring out how to make sure your and your baby's needs are covered with the income or incomes you expect to have. What if something happens to you or your partner and that income disappears?

The answer, of course, is life insurance. It's possible one or both of you already have some through your jobs. Hopefully, you have some kind of disability coverage as well. Check with your employer to see what coverage you have and whether you can or should increase it.

Otherwise, you'll need to think about buying your own insurance. There are a lot of options, so again, you'll need to do some research and get some expert advice.

If one of you will be staying home with the baby and not working for pay, don't make the mistake of thinking you only need to consider insurance for the working partner. The work the stay-at-home partner does also has monetary value, something that becomes crystal clear when you add up what it would cost if you had to hire full-time child and household help.

Certainly, the loss of either of you would be catastrophic, and a financial payout wouldn't make that loss any less painful. The point of having life insurance is to make sure whoever is left behind isn't devastated financially as well as emotionally.

## *Wills and advance directives*

On a similar topic, if you and your partner haven't made up wills and advance directives, now is the time.

You and your partner need wills, even if you're not wealthy. Chances are you have something of value to leave behind, whether it's cash, real estate or a comic book collection. A will can cover so much more than dispersal of your worldly goods, though.

If something were to happen to both of you, who would you want to raise your child? If you haven't designated someone in your will, the state will likely take him or her into care and make that decision for you.

What do you want to happen to your social media accounts if you die? Your will can include your user names and passwords, along with instructions on saving your online content and deactivating accounts (or not). If you want to be very thorough you can even leave messages to be posted after your death, although there's a fine line here between being thoughtful and just being creepy.

## *Health insurance*

Ideally, one or both of you will have health insurance that is subsidized by an employer, and that insurance will cover pregnancy and childbirth. Perhaps you have coverage through your state that is based on a limited income or has been able to get coverage on a sliding scale. Otherwise, you may have been paying high premiums for policies that don't cover much or even going without.

It's best to have health insurance in place before getting pregnant, as to whether pregnancy can be considered a pre-existing condition for insurance purposes is subject to change. Depending on when and where your partner becomes pregnant, insurers might be able to charge higher premiums or even refuse to insure her.

If you haven't checked your health coverage before now, do it right away. See if your partner is, or can be, added to your policy, or if she has one of her own. Your insurance plan may have a specified open enrollment period during which coverage changes can be made, but pregnancy is usually considered a reason to allow changes outside the enrollment period. Check the pregnancy and childbirth benefits to see what's covered. You'll need to plan for any gaps in coverage.

If your partner doesn't have health insurance and can't find affordable coverage, she may qualify under state-based Medicaid and Children's Health Insurance Program (CHIP). These programs have income requirements and vary from state to state.

# Chapter 6:

# Preparing your home

## *Where will the baby sleep?*

It's a very good idea to talk with your partner about where the baby is going to sleep while keeping in mind that whatever you decide, your feelings may change over time.

Options include a crib, a bassinet, a bassinet attached to your bed, and in the bed with you. Every possibility has its fans and its detractors, and you may be surprised at how strongly some of your friends and family feel about them. The decision about where your baby is going to sleep is deeply personal and should be decided by you and your partner.

If you are setting up a separate room, or nursery, for the baby, you'll have lots of choices as far as materials, colors, and lighting.

## *Crib*

A crib is the default choice for most parents. A new crib can be expensive and you'll only use it for two or three years at most (less if your child is a precocious climber). You might be offered someone else's old crib or be tempted to buy a used one; if you are, make sure it meets current safety recommendations. Too much space between the bars or between the bottom and side of the crib can trap a baby's body or head, with tragic consequences.

## *Bassinet*

A bassinet is a small cradle-like bed or basket that a baby can sleep in until they are old enough to sit up on their own, around six months or so. At that point, the bassinet won't be big enough or stable enough to hold them.

## *Co-sleeper bassinet*

A co-sleeper is a bassinet that fits against the side of your bed. It's a compromise that keeps baby safely in his or her own space, but reassuringly close. It's also possible to "sidecar" a crib by leaving one side off of it and attaching it securely to your bed. Care must be taken to ensure there's no space between bassinet or crib and bed where the baby could get trapped.

## *In bed with you*

Referred to as co-sleeping or the family bed, keeping your baby in your bed with you may be the most natural option; families have been sleeping together for as long as there have been families. There are many advantages to co-sleeping, and some disadvantages as well. Co-sleeping can enhance bonding with the baby and be especially convenient for breastfeeding; while you won't necessarily get to sleep through the night, you can at least avoid having to get out of bed to attend to diapering or feeding.

On the other hand, co-sleeping may be dangerous for the baby if either you or your partner are big people, heavy sleepers or under the influence of intoxicants or pain medications. And of course, having a baby in the bed changes the dynamic between you and your partner. It's hard to spoon or cuddle with a little body between you. And when you're both ready to start having sex again, a little creativity will be needed if the bed is your usual spot for intimacy.

If you do decide on co-sleeping, it's a good idea to talk about how long you both think you'll want to continue. You may find you love the family bed more than you thought you would, or you may tire of it sooner than expected. And your partner may feel the same—or the opposite! As with so many issues you'll face as parents, it's important to keep the lines of communication open and to take care of your relationship just as you take care of your child.

## *How much gear do you really need?*

The variety and magnitude of gear for use at home and away is astounding. What you end up with is limited only by your imagination, budget, and available space. A reasonable list includes:

- **Crib**: bassinet or other space for baby to sleep.
- **Blankets**: You'll want quite a few of the small, light blankets known commonly called receiving blankets. You'll use them for everything from swaddling the baby to protecting your clothing from spit-up. And there will be lots of spit-ups.
- **Infant car seat**: Most are now designed to accommodate the safety needs of little ones from newborn to

toddler. Be wary of used car seats, as it isn't all that uncommon for them to be recalled due to safety issues. Make sure you understand exactly how to secure the seat in your car; practice taking it out and buckling it back in well before your baby is due.

- **Diapers and wipes or washcloths**: Lots of them. You can't even imagine how many diapers you'll go through. There's no doubt disposable diapers are the easiest to deal with, but they do create an enormous landfill burden. Biodegradable diapers are available, but they're not cheap. Cloth diapers can live forever as rags after your baby outgrows them, but they can be a lot of work, and some argue the frequent laundering and disinfection they require isn't a lot greener in the long run. Diaper services that pick up dirty diapers and drop off clean ones may be available.

- **Seasonally appropriate clothing**: Babies aren't very adept at regulating their body temperature for the first year or two. They can easily get overheated if they are overdressed, or become hypothermic if they are underdressed.
- **Stroller**: There are two basic kinds of stroller, the kind that's like a

bassinet on wheels, and the kind that is super light and foldable. The first kind lets you carry lots of gear, traverse uneven terrain and protect the baby from sun, wind, and rain. The second kind, often called an umbrella stroller, is way less fancy but is easy to pack up and take along. The ideal solution is to have one of each.

## *Maintaining a healthy environment*

### *Drugs and alcohol*

Once your baby is crawling, keeping intoxicants out of reach will obviously be an issue. Until then, the concern is passive exposure and the danger of being cared for by adults who are under the influence. Exposing a baby to second-hand smoke from the pot, crack or meth, or breastfeeding after using any drug, are forms of child abuse, plain and simple. A baby's safety and wellbeing require parents and caregivers to be present, alert and aware of what's happening around them.

*Tobacco*

There's no amount of second-hand tobacco smoke that is safe for a baby. Even limited exposure can contribute to asthma, ear and respiratory infections and even sudden infant death syndrome (SIDS). Smoking inside the home is obviously off-limits. Vaping is clearly safer than smoking cigarettes, but that doesn't mean it's safe in your home. You'll still take in toxic amounts of nicotine and other chemicals, and the particulate matter you puff out can still be breathed in by those around you. If either you or your partner is dependent on the nicotine in any smoky or vaporous form, now you have a really good reason to quit.

*Pets*

Besides the emotional benefits of growing up with a beloved pet, research suggests early exposure to furry family members can help prevent a child from developing allergies and asthma. Safety comes first, though. Experts recommend making sure you can control your dog with voice commands, and get it used to baby smells and sounds long before you bring that fragrant little sound machine home. Some dogs will see a newborn as a kind of hairless puppy, while others will see potential prey. Make sure you know which kind of dog you have. The advice for is the same for cats (except for the part about obeying voice commands, of course).

If you have a cat that goes outside and also uses a litter box inside, there are special concerns when your partner is pregnant. If your partner contracts toxoplasmosis while she's pregnant, the parasite can damage the baby's eyes and brain. Toxoplasmosis is a parasite cats pick up by eating infected small animals. The cat then excretes oocysts, which are kind of like tough little eggs, in their feces. Humans become infected by inhaling or swallowing the oocysts. This is obviously a concern with litter boxes, but it can also be a problem if cats use your yard or garden as a toilet.

It's best if your partner avoids scooping the litter box while pregnant; if it's unavoidable she should wear gloves and wash her hands afterward.

# Chapter 7:
# First trimester — Conception through 12 weeks

For convenience, pregnancy is divided into trimesters, or three periods each lasting three calendar months. Together they make up the familiar nine-month pregnancy.

An obstetrician or midwife looks at it a little differently, though. Medically, the average full-term pregnancy lasts 40 weeks. This is counted from the first day of the woman's last menstrual period. If she has a textbook menstrual cycle, she'll have ovulated two weeks after her last period started, and conception will have happened around then. This means that by the time the fertilized egg settles into her uterus, she is already considered to be two weeks pregnant. (Calculations can be more complicated if the egg was fertilized outside your partner's body and implanted into her uterus as an embryo. In this case, your care team will explain how dates will be calculated.)

This calculation helps estimate a due date, or date the baby is expected to be born. The emphasis here is on *expected*—and we know what happens to expectations when it comes to having a baby! The expected due date (EDD) may change as the baby grows and it gets easier to see just how far along it is.

The first trimester can be a little rocky. First, there's the joy (or shock) of finding out your partner is pregnant. Then, as her body starts swinging into the baby-making mode, the rising tide of hormones makes itself felt. Certain discomforts are very common in the first trimester, and your partner is likely to experience a few.

## *What the first trimester feels like*

### *Morning sickness*

Most women will have it, but the severity varies. Because hCG, the pregnancy hormone blamed for so many early discomforts, is made by the placenta, morning sickness can be taken as a sign of a healthy placenta that will be part of a healthy pregnancy. Multiple pregnancies (twins, triplets or more) involve multiple placentas, and so morning sickness may be more severe.

Although it tends to be worse in the morning when she wakes up with an empty stomach, morning sickness can occur any time of day. Eating saltine crackers or some similarly bland snack before getting out of bed may help. Ice cubes, popsicles, frequent small meals and ginger supplements or tea throughout the day are other popular treatments.

A less common and more severe form of morning sickness known as hyperemesis gravidarum may require medical care. Hyperemesis means severe vomiting, and it's hard for the woman who suffers it to take in the nutrients she and the baby both need. She may need medication to calm the vomiting, and really bad cases sometimes call for hospitalization. Fortunately, this is rare.

## *Tender breasts*

As much as they are valued for other reasons, breasts are built to feed babies. In the months to come her breasts will get larger and heavier as they get ready for their star turn. Early in pregnancy, their heightened state of alert may cause them to become exquisitely tender, especially the nipples. She'll be most comfortable in a close-fitting bra that reduces movement and friction. Don't be surprised to find her wearing one to bed, and don't take it personally if she doesn't want you touching her breasts—at all.

*Fatigue*

Hormone levels aren't all that's changing in the first trimester. Blood pressure, blood sugar levels, and moods may fluctuate as well. Your partner may need more sleep and have less stamina for physical exertion than she normally does. If she has a full-time job she may find it hard to get through her work day and may feel exhausted by the time she gets home.

Remember this is common in the first trimester and she will most likely feel more like herself in a few weeks. Show your support by taking up the slack around the house and encouraging her to rest.

### *Frequent urination*

Later on, she'll need to pee a lot because her increased blood volume is kicking her kidneys into overdrive and because the growing baby is pressing on her bladder. In the first trimester, she may feel the need to go a lot because of—you guessed it—hormones.

### *Sensitivity to tastes and smells*

The old TV trope about pregnant women craving pickles and ice cream or some other odd food combination has some basis in fact. She may be repelled by foods she normally loves for reasons she can't really explain, and find that what really hits the spot is something she doesn't usually eat. Overall, of course, the goal is a healthy diet for a healthy pregnancy, but it's fine to indulge her cravings within reason. This is especially true if she also has morning sickness and it's a challenge to get anything down at all.

*Headaches*

Not every woman will have headaches in the first trimester. For those who do, they may range from mild to migraine. Regular meals and adequate fluids will help prevent headaches caused by low blood sugar or dehydration, although this can be tricky if she has the kind of morning sickness that lasts all day. Headaches can also be a problem if she is trying to cut back on her usual caffeine intake. It's generally a good idea to avoid unnecessary medications in the first trimester when the baby's organs and other parts are forming, but that doesn't mean mom has to suffer. If her headaches are distressing, encourage her to talk to her doctor or midwife about how she can treat them safely.

## *Prenatal care*

Prenatal care covers everything from thinking about getting pregnant to the arrival of the baby. Ideally, your partner will have met with a healthcare provider before getting pregnant, but this may not have happened if she's uninsured or if the pregnancy was a surprise. Otherwise, the first prenatal appointment is usually booked for about eight weeks from the first day of her last period.

If your partner doesn't have health insurance, your local Planned Parenthood clinic is a good place to start looking for prenatal care. She may be able to get all her prenatal care there, either free or at a reduced cost. They can also help her find out if she qualifies for health insurance through your state of residence or if there are other affordable health services available.

The first prenatal visit is usually the most comprehensive and will involve a complete health history, physical examination, and blood tests. The information gathered will form a baseline that future visits will build on.

After the first visit, a typical timeline for a normal, healthy first pregnancy will include prenatal visits every four weeks for the first 28 weeks, then every two weeks until 36 weeks, and then once a week until the baby comes. Your partner's actual schedule may vary, depending on whether it's her first baby and whether she has, or develops, any health problems.

If it's too early to hear the baby's heartbeat with a handheld Doppler at the first prenatal visit, it will certainly be heard by the second one. First trimester ultrasounds are not routinely done but may be recommended if a problem is suspected or if it's important to determine just how far along the pregnancy is.

## *First-trimester screen*

Your partner may be offered a combination test known as the first-trimester screen. In the first part of the test, her blood is tested for substances that might indicate the baby has Down syndrome or certain other uncommon chromosomal abnormalities. The second part of the test is an ultrasound that measures tissue at the back of the baby's neck. Taken together, these two tests make it possible to estimate the *risk* of an abnormality, not the presence of an abnormality. If the screen suggests there is a medium to high risk, more testing can be done.

## *The awkward bits*

### *Vaginal odor*

Changes in hormone levels and vaginal pH may cause your partner's odor to be stronger, or just different, than usual. It may even smell something like what she had to eat for lunch. This is perfectly normal. A strong fishy odor though may be a symptom of a bacterial infection that needs attention. You can try to find a gentle way to alert your partner if you think her smell is abnormal, but with her increased sensitivity to odors she probably already knows.

## *Gas and constipation*

The hormones of pregnancy tend to cause muscles to relax. The GI system relies on muscular contractions to keep food moving as it's digested, and it can slow down a bit in pregnancy. The result is often constipation, bloating and gassiness. Gas is released as bacteria in the intestines break down nutrients, so the longer it takes for the nutrients to move through, the more gas can be produced. The anus is, of course, part of the GI system, and holding in gas requires a tightening of anal muscles. As those muscles soften, your partner may be dismayed to discover her farts taking on a life of their own, popping out at the most inopportune moments. Do your best to laugh with her, not at her.

## *Stress incontinence*

In the last trimester, especially, the weight of the growing baby will press against your partner's bladder. Not only will she need to pee a lot, but she may also find that anything that increases pressure in her abdomen—like sneezing, for example—may cause urine to leak right out. This is called stress incontinence. If this happens to her she might want to wear panty liners.

## *Facial hair*

Your partner may find something growing in the pregnancy she definitely didn't count on: a beard. In fact, she may notice new hair on other parts of her body as well, including on her belly and around her nipples. This is partly due to new hair growth, partly to hair growing in a bit darker than usual, and partly to hairs not falling out as they normally would. All of this is perfectly normal and temporary.

## *Hemorrhoids*

Hemorrhoids are swollen veins in the rectum and around the anus. They are a very common discomfort of pregnancy. Early on they may be caused by constipation, and later by the increased pressure of an abdomen full of baby. They may also result from, or be made worse by, the strain of pushing the baby out. The best defense against hemorrhoids is to prevent constipation by taking in lots of fiber and fluids, getting regular exercise and going to the bathroom as soon as the need arises (rather than holding it for a more convenient time).

### *Leaking breasts*

Long before the baby comes, your partner's breasts may begin producing a thick, creamy fluid called colostrum. It will take a few days after the baby is born for her breasts to fill with milk, and the colostrum will tide the baby over until they do. Not every woman will leak like this during pregnancy. If your partner does, she may want to wear breast pads, or nursing pads, inside her bra. They will come in handy after the baby comes, too, as it isn't uncommon for a nursing mother's breasts to leak milk when they're full or even when she hears a baby cry.

# Chapter 8:

# Second trimester — *13 to 27 weeks*

For many women, the second trimester is the most enjoyable part of pregnancy. Morning sickness resolves, her energy returns, she starts feeling the baby move and everything seems to be falling into place. Or not.

## *Physical changes*

The second trimester is when your partner is likely to start really looking and feeling pregnant. Her growing bump is not the only noticeable change, though. While every woman is an individual and every pregnancy is unique, there are some features that are common to this stage.

## *Melasma*

Melanin is the brown pigment that determines skin color. Exposure to the sun causes an increase in melanin, but pregnancy hormones can stimulate melanin production too. Melasma is sometimes called the "mask of pregnancy" because it is seen so commonly on the faces of pregnant women. It shows up even on women whose skin is naturally rich in melanin. The downside to melasma is that it tends to be patchy and uneven. The good news is that it should fully resolve after the baby comes. In the meantime, your partner should be sure to use a good, broad-spectrum sunscreen with an SPF of at least 30 whenever she's in the sun.

## *Linea Negra*

This is a dark line, sometimes called the pregnancy line, on a pregnant woman's abdomen that runs from the belly button down to the pubic bone. Sometimes it extends above the belly button to the ribs. It's another instance of increased melanin production that usually resolves after the baby is born, although it may take a few months to disappear completely.

## *Stretch marks*

Whether your partner gets stretch marks, and how pronounced they are, depends partly on genetics and partly on how much weight she gains, and how quickly. They may develop on her belly, breasts, thighs or buttocks and are due to tearing of connective tissue under the skin. Stretch marks usually look red or purple during pregnancy and fade in color afterward, although they never actually go away. The stretching skin over her belly is likely to be itchy, too. Although there's no science behind claims that coconut butter or other salves will prevent stretch marks, keeping the skin well-moisturized may help with the itching.

### *Braxton Hicks contractions*

These "practice" contractions usually kick in during the second trimester, becoming more intense in the third. Your partner will notice her belly becoming tighter and then relaxing, occasionally at first and more frequently as time goes on. It's possible she will find them startling or uncomfortable; some women like to visualize them as giving the baby a big hug. Braxton Hicks contractions don't open the cervix and are not a sign of early labor, but your partner should definitely check in with her doctor or midwife if she's worried.

### *Round ligament pain*

As her belly grows and gets heavier, your partner may sometimes have sharp pains in her groin, usually to one side or the other (or both), rather than in the middle. The pain is due to pressure on, and spasming of, the round ligaments that support the uterus. She may experience stabbing pains when she changes position suddenly, such as when rolling over and sitting up in bed, or when coughing or sneezing. She may not be able to avoid round ligament pain altogether, but changing position more slowly and gently may help.

### *Fetal movement*

Sometime during the second trimester, your partner will start feeling the baby move. The first time may be sudden like it is on TV. It is more likely, though, that she will gradually become aware that what she thought were just more gas bubbles moving through her intestines are actually kicks and pokes from her little passenger. Traditionally the onset of noticeable fetal movement was known as "quickening"—ie, the beginning of life.

People often refer to the fetal movement as "kicking" but the baby does much more than a kick in there. As it grows it will sometimes feel like it's doing Tai Kwon Do, and it will, in fact, do gymnastics, including somersaults. In time you'll be able to feel the movements by putting your hand on her belly, and eventually, you'll be able to see them. You may even get to where you can confidently identify a moving part as a foot or an elbow!

## *Libido*

First trimester discomforts may have resolved, but hormones are still running high. Your partner may feel very sexy, the most extreme opposite of sexy, or something in between. Creating life is probably the most intimate thing two people can do together, and you may find your lovemaking increasingly tender and loving. If you're not on the same page sexually, though, there's plenty of opportunity for conflict and resentment. Maybe you find her more beautiful and desirable than ever, but she pushes you away. Maybe her libido is at a peak but you can't help feeling weird about having sex with a baby on board. This is another opportunity to practice open, honest communication that will help get you through the coming challenges of parenthood.

## *Prenatal care*

During the second trimester, your partner will probably see her healthcare provider about every four weeks.

### *Fundal height*

During these visits, the healthcare provider will measure the distance from your partner's pubic bone to the top of her uterus, known as the fundal height. This is done to estimate the baby's size and how it compares to how far along in pregnancy your partner is thought to be.

After 20 weeks the fundal height in centimeters is expected to match the number of weeks of pregnancy, so for example, at 25 weeks the fundal height should be 25 centimeters. Fundal height is a convenient guide to fetal growth but not always 100 percent accurate. If there are any concerns about the baby's size or whether the due date has been estimated correctly, an ultrasound will probably be ordered.

### *Fetal heartbeat*

Listening to the baby's heartbeat with the handheld Doppler is often the highlight of second-trimester visits, even if you've heard it before. It's the reassurance that your baby is doing well and may help you, the dad, feel more connected to him or her.

### *Ultrasound*

While they aren't really necessary for normal pregnancies, ultrasounds have become very common. If your partner hasn't already had one it's likely to be offered now, and that peek into the baby's hidden world is hard to resist. It may be possible to determine the gender by this point, so you should decide beforehand whether or not you want to know. Ultrasounds can be hard to decipher and it's possible only the technician will be able to tell for sure, but sometimes it's pretty obvious, especially if you get a 3D ultrasound. Of course, the medical rationale for ultrasound is to make sure everything is okay, and so measurements will be taken and limbs and organs will be inspected to make sure there aren't any obvious problems.

## *Urine test*

On each prenatal visit, your partner will be asked to provide a urine sample to check for gestational diabetes (sugar in the urine), preeclampsia (protein in the urine) and urinary tract infection (white blood cells in the urine). This is usually done by dipping a testing strip into the sample, and in some offices, your partner will be able to do this herself.

## *Weight*

Your partner's weight will be checked at every visit to make sure she's gaining at a healthy rate. If she was underweight or had a healthy BMI when she got pregnant, she'll be expected to gain about a pound a week during the second trimester. Some of this is the baby, but most of it is a combination of body fat, amniotic fluid and increased blood volume. If she started out with a high BMI, her goal will be to gain about half a pound per week.

## *Genetic testing*

Testing for genetic abnormalities may be offered during the second trimester, especially if either you or your partner are known to carry a genetic condition, or if there are any conditions that run in either of your families. A quad test, or quad marker screen, checks for substances in your partner's blood that might indicate the baby has problems with the brain or spinal cord or has Down syndrome or another chromosomal abnormality. Like the first trimester screen, the quad test measures the *risk* of abnormality, not the presence of abnormality. A calculated risk that is medium or high can be confirmed with ultrasound and amniocentesis.

## *Amniocentesis*

Amniocentesis involves inserting a needle into the uterus and withdrawing some of the amniotic fluid the baby is floating in. Genetic testing can be done on cells from the baby that are found in the amniotic fluid. Amniocentesis is highly accurate and can screen for a number of conditions that can't be diagnosed before birth by any other means. It does carry a small risk of miscarriage, though, and an even smaller risk of infection or early labor.

Amniocentesis is strictly optional, and if it's offered or recommended you and your partner will need to weigh the risks and benefits before deciding if you want to go through with it. Knowing about a problem can give you time to get ready for a baby that will have special needs, or to consider terminating the pregnancy if the problems are very severe.

# Chapter 9:
# Third trimester — *28 to 40 weeks*

The third trimester is when pregnancy and the fact that a baby is on the way becomes obvious and real. The seventh month is when your partner's bump blossoms, especially if this is her first baby. It may be hard to believe it's going to get even bigger over the next two months!

After feeling cheerful and energetic during the second trimester, she may now start slowing down and facing some new discomforts. All of this is balanced, of course, with the excitement and anticipation of the baby's arrival—the big payoff for all this hard work.

By 28 weeks the baby's parts are all built and refined, and now all that's left is to grow, fill out and generally get ready for life outside the womb. This can be a joyous and busy time for you and your partner and a time that brings its own challenges.

## *The baby bump*

Up until now, the changes in your partner's body may have been somewhat subtle. Yes, her belly rounded and she may have added some extra padding elsewhere, but the changes might not have been pregnancy-specific. From here on out, they will be much more so.

The size, weight, and shape of her belly will begin to change her center of gravity. Ligaments in her pelvis are also softening and loosening, and she may start to walk and move very differently.

If you have access to an empathy or sympathy belly, it will help give you some insight into what your partner is experiencing. An empathy belly is a weighted vest that gives you an idea of what it feels like to carry the size and weight of a pregnant belly and breasts. You may not be likely to have one lying around, but you'll probably get a chance to try one out in your childbirth preparation classes.

### *Belly bands and support belts*

The female pelvis is wider than the male pelvis, with a larger opening in the center, perfect for passing a baby through. Except, have you seen the size of a newborn baby? Have you ever looked at your partner and wondered how on earth that's going to work?

Part of the answer lies in the changes that take place in the pelvis in the last trimester. The pelvis isn't just one solid piece; it has joints, and ligaments holding the joints together. In pregnancy the ligaments get looser, allowing some remodeling of the pelvis. This is good news when it's time to birth that baby, but in the meantime, it can cause some discomfort.

The pressure of the baby on stretched ligaments can cause pain in the pelvis, groin, and back. One way to help ease this discomfort is to wear a belly band or maternity support belt. There are many different designs, but they are kind of first cousins to the support belts worn for hernias and heavy lifting. Basically, a belly band or belt goes around the back and under the belly, supporting it and relieving ligament strain.

## *Sleeping position*

Your partner may have been advised not to sleep on her back during the last trimester. This is because the weight of the baby can compress the vena cava, a large blood vessel that runs under the uterus. Squeezing the vena cava can cause her blood pressure to drop. In theory, this low blood pressure can cause her to feel dizzy and nauseated and possibly deprive the baby of needed oxygen. The science doesn't really back this up, though, and if your partner finds she only sleeps well on her back she probably doesn't need to worry about it. She can always clear it with her doctor or midwife, just to be sure. It's also possible that she'll find sleeping on her back impossible anyway, as pressure on her diaphragm can make it hard to breathe. She may sleep much better on her side, especially with lots of pillows to tuck around her belly and between her legs.

### *Pregnancy brain*

Yes, this is a real thing. Feeling spacey and forgetful in the third trimester is reassuringly common. Your partner may need lots of notes and lists to help navigate her daily life, whether it's reminding her of an appointment she has made, or even why she walked into that room. This is due in part to hormones, of course—isn't everything at this point?—but there are other factors at play as well. Her growing belly, weird dreams and need to pee during the night may be causing some sleep deprivation. Having so much to do before the baby arrives may be stressing her out, and stress makes everyone forgetful. And finally, she is likely becoming preoccupied with thoughts of childbirth and caring for a newborn. One theory is that losing focus on other things and thinking more about the baby is just what nature intends. In any case, pregnancy brain is a temporary disability.

### *Increased blood volume*

To meet the demands of building a new human, your partner's total blood volume has by now increased by 50 percent or about 1250 ml. That's 42 ounces, or more than five cups. This is great for the baby, but all that extra fluid can have some unpleasant side effects for mom. She may notice swelling of her fingers, toes, feet and ankles. She may develop varicose veins in her legs, and her nose may feel stuffy. And of course, there's the frequent need to pee, which is partially due to the babysitting on her bladder but also to her kidneys processing all that extra fluid. She should talk with her doctor or midwife about appropriate comfort measures and treatment options, which may include support stockings, saltwater nasal rinses, elevating her feet and removing jewelry, especially rings.

## *Activity*

Many women stay very active right up until they go into labor, whether because they want to or because they have no choice—the world doesn't stop and wait for your baby to come, after all. If your partner was athletic before getting pregnant and hasn't faced any unexpected complications, she may keep up her usual pace and feel quite comfortable doing so. Even so, no woman completely escapes the physical reality of late pregnancy.

### *Kick counting*

By the third trimester, your partner should be feeling the baby move quite regularly. By 30 weeks she'll want to start paying attention to just how often she feels movement. In addition to her general awareness of the baby's activity, she may be advised to have a couple of times each day when she actually counts how many times in an hour the baby moves.

We tend to talk about the baby "kicking," and sometimes it does feel like feet are flying, but that's not all that's going on. Most babies don't settle into one position until just before labor begins; until then, they move in every direction and at any given moment may be upside down, right side up or lying sideways. They may face outward, toward mom's spine or off to the side.

Whatever is going on in there, some kind of activity should be felt at least six times per hour. Your partner will likely be advised to set aside a couple of times each day for kick counting, in which she should sit quietly and count the number of movements she feels. Babies in the womb do sleep and will have quiet times, but your partner should check in with her doctor or midwife if she's feeling less movement than expected.

## *Physical preparation*

A baby carried to term is going to be born one way or another, whether you and your partner prepare or not. If she's planning to deliver vaginally (the old school way), though, there are some things she can do to get in shape for the big event. There's even something you can help with.

### *Kegel exercises*

Kegels can be tedious, but doing them doesn't just help your partner prepare for childbirth; it also helps her get back into shape afterward. Kegels work the pelvic floor muscles that support the uterus, bladder, and intestines.

Keeping these muscles strong will help her do the hard work of childbirth and also help her bounce back afterward.

Men also have pelvic floor muscles, and doing Kegels can help treat and prevent dribbling and erectile dysfunction. Kegel time can be couple time!

To activate the right muscles, pretend you are trying to hold in urine or gas. Squeeze for a count of five and release. Three sets of 10 reps per day are ideal, both for you and for your partner.

## *Perineal massage*

The perineum is the space between the vagina and the anus (or in your case, between the scrotum and the anus). Women are often advised to spend some time massaging and stretching their perineum before giving birth for the first time. The hope is that this will help keep the perineum, which can tear or be cut to make more room for the baby to emerge, intact. Studies haven't found really strong evidence perineal massage works, but it can't hurt.

It's generally recommended to place two lubricated fingers partway into the vagina and apply firm but gentle pressure, first downward toward the anus and then to each side. It's easier for you to do this than for your partner to do it for herself, especially late in pregnancy when she may have trouble reaching that far at all. She should check with her doctor or midwife first to make sure there's no reason she should avoid perineal massage.

## *Childbirth preparation classes*

Childbirth classes are usually planned to begin around six or seven months into pregnancy. They can be scheduled later, but there's always the chance your baby will surprise you with an early appearance, leaving you unprepared.

Traditionally, classes are offered through, and usually at, the facility where you're planning to have the baby. If that's a hospital or birthing center, classes are likely to include a tour of the labor and delivery areas. If you're planning a home birth, classes may be offered with a midwife, birth assistant or doula, and the location will vary.

Nowadays there are many ways to approach childbirth preparation. Many of the places that offer classes in a series also offer "express" preparation that fits everything into one class. And of course, there are video and live-streamed online classes.

Classes can include everything from fetal development to childbirth to newborn care or can be broken down into separate classes for each topic. They may focus on one particular approach to childbirth, such as Lamaze or the Bradley method, or they may touch on aspects of many.

The kind of preparation you and your partner choose will depend on your previous experience and knowledge base, your schedules and learning styles, and the kind of birth you hope to have.

## *Making a birth plan*

A birth plan is a very epitome of hoping for the

best and planning for the worst. You and your partner should think about how you want the delivery to go, and also how you want to respond if things don't go according to plan. You should write your plan out, give a copy to the doctor or midwife and to the birth assistant or doula if you have one, and pack a copy in with your birth kit or go-bag.

You can get a birth plan template from a healthcare provider or find one online. You can make it as simple or as comprehensive as you like, covering everything from whether your partner wants an epidural to what music she wants to have to play while she's in labor to whether you will allow the baby to be bathed.

Just keep in mind that circumstances may not allow everything to play out the way you plan, and your partner may change her mind as labor progresses. She might find she wants a different playlist (or no music at all), or be surprised by which comfort measures actually help the most. If she wants to avoid an epidural or other pain medication, she needs to think about how important this is to her—if she finds herself wanting something for pain after all, does she want you to agree, or try to talk her out of it?

Just keep in mind a birth plan is more of a wish list than a recipe. Surprises, whether large or small, are inevitable.

## What the baby's doing

### The baby drops

The ideal position for a baby to be in before labor begins is head down, facing mom's spine.

There's some maneuvering to be done when it's time to slip under the pubic bone on the way to the birth canal, and being oriented this way is best. At some point before labor begins, either just before or even weeks before, most babies will drop lower into mom's pelvis and settle into this head-down position. Less commonly a baby settles in right side up, or breech.

A traditional term for this settling is lightening because the woman often feels much lighter in her upper abdomen as space increases for her stomach and diaphragm. She may breathe easier and have relief from indigestion and heartburn. At the same time, though, she may feel much more pressure lower down, aggravating hemorrhoids, decreasing her bladder capacity and sometimes even making walking awkward. This change in the baby's position is also known as dropping or engaging.

# Chapter 10:

# Complications in pregnancy

The best defense against complications in pregnancy is a healthy lifestyle and good prenatal care. But complications can arise and may be due to factors completely out of your and your partner's control.

Some of these complications are pretty scary. It's good to be aware of symptoms that need attention, but also to remember you probably won't be dealing with any of the really serious ones.

## *Miscarriage*

One or two out of every 10 confirmed pregnancies will end in miscarriage, usually within the first trimester. It's something to be aware of, but not to spend a lot of time worrying about. Remember, this means eight to nine out of every 10 confirmed pregnancies carry on and result in a baby.

In most cases, the reason for an early miscarriage is never known. It will usually be assumed there was a problem with that particular pregnancy that kept it from developing further. For most women, miscarriage is a one-off. It may cause some anxiety the next time around, but it's overwhelmingly likely it won't happen again.

A very small number of women do go on to have a second or even a third early pregnancy loss. This is known as recurrent miscarriage.

After a third miscarriage, an investigation into what's causing this to happen is likely to be done. A cause isn't always found, though, and even women who have had recurrent miscarriages more often than not go on to have successful pregnancies.

## *Symptoms*

Miscarriage sometimes happens in real life the way it does on TV, but usually, it does not. Rather than a dramatic event with sudden severe pain and heavy bleeding, the end of early pregnancy is likely to sneak up on you. In fact, the first sign of an impending miscarriage may be that your partner suddenly feels much better. As hormone levels fall she may celebrate the end of morning sickness and the other early discomforts.

Later, cramping and spotting make it clear the pregnancy is in trouble.

At this point, she will most likely be sent in for an ultrasound to determine "fetal viability," that is, whether or not the fetus is still alive. If it is not, decisions will need to be made about how to proceed.

In most cases, she will be sent home, possibly with something to take for pain. Depending on how far along she was, she may experience something like a normal or severe period, or even something more like labor pains, because her cervix must dilate to allow the uterine contents to pass. This may take hours or days. She may pass blood clots and indistinct tissue, or even a recognizable fetus. If that happens, you'll need to think about what you want to do with the remains. How to say goodbye to a much-hoped-for baby is a very personal decision.

*Complications*

Bleeding may continue for a few days, much like a regular period. Heavy bleeding, bleeding for more than a few days, foul-smelling discharge, fever or flu-like symptoms require medical care. It isn't common but sometimes tissue remains in the uterus, leading to what is known as an incomplete miscarriage. This can cause heavy bleeding and infection, and sometimes a procedure is needed to remove what's been left behind.

# Ectopic pregnancy

Conception—the meeting of the egg and the

sperm—takes place in the fallopian tubes, the very narrow channels eggs pass through when they leave the ovaries. In a normal pregnancy, the fertilized egg continues along until it reaches the uterus and settles in.

In an ectopic pregnancy, the egg settles in somewhere other than the uterus, usually the fallopian tube itself. Less common spots include the ovary and the cervix. Because there's a tiny space between the fallopian tubes and the ovaries, in very rare cases a fertilized egg may escape the reproductive system altogether and travel out into the abdomen.

An ectopic pregnancy is not a normal pregnancy, and a woman who has one may or may not have typical symptoms of early pregnancy. Whether she feels pregnant or not, at some point she will start noticing pain in her pelvis that is definitely different from menstrual cramps, and she may have some vaginal bleeding.

An ectopic pregnancy in a fallopian tube, also known as a tubal pregnancy, may grow large enough to rupture the tube, causing severe pain and bleeding. Sometimes an ectopic pregnancy bleeds internally. When this happens, she may feel intense pressure in her rectum and lower abdomen, have shooting pain up into her back and shoulders and feel dizzy and lightheaded. A ruptured ectopic pregnancy is a medical emergency and can be life-threatening.

There is no way to save an ectopic pregnancy, and it can never result in a baby. Once your partner is out of physical danger, grieving over the loss of the pregnancy is likely to begin. If the fallopian tube was damaged beyond repair it will be harder to conceive again, and this may add to the emotional toll.

## *Hydatiform mole*

It is very unlikely your partner will have a hydatiform mole, also known as molar pregnancy, as they are pretty rare. Like an ectopic pregnancy, a molar pregnancy will not result in a baby.

A hydatiform mole grows from tissue that would form the placenta in a normal pregnancy. In a complete molar pregnancy, an egg is fertilized by the father's sperm but for some reason, the mother's share of DNA is missing. In a partial molar pregnancy, the mother's DNA is present but there are two copies of the father's

DNA, possibly because the egg has been fertilized by two sperm.

In a complete molar pregnancy, no embryo is formed at all. In a partial molar pregnancy, the embryo may begin to form but won't be viable and will eventually miscarry. In rare cases, a molar pregnancy may grow from tissue left behind after a miscarriage or normal delivery. Even more rarely, a molar pregnancy can turn cancerous.

A molar pregnancy may start out just like a normal pregnancy but usually grows much faster. Instead of a slow-growing baby bump, a woman may suddenly look very pregnant very early on. She is likely to have bleeding and severe morning sickness as well. A molar pregnancy is an uncommon but serious complication that requires immediate medical attention.

## *Hyperemesis gravidarum*

More than just severe morning sickness, hyperemesis gravidarum is severe nausea and vomiting in pregnancy that causes weight loss, dehydration and electrolyte imbalances. It can make it impossible for the woman to take in the nutrients she and the baby need and can affect her kidneys, liver and thyroid function.

Sometimes hyperemesis can be managed with comfort measures at home. Sometimes IV fluids are needed to replace body fluids lost through vomiting and being unable to drink water. In extreme cases, a woman may have to be hospitalized and liquid nutrition delivered through an IV or stomach tube. As a last resort, the pregnancy may have to be terminated.

## *Gestational diabetes*

You may be familiar with diabetes. Type I is the kind where your pancreas doesn't produce enough insulin. Insulin is needed to move glucose, or sugar, from the blood into cells, where it's used for energy. Without insulin, glucose builds up in the blood and cells are starved for energy. A person with Type I diabetes has to inject insulin.

Type II diabetes, which is becoming increasingly common in the US, is the kind where you produce insulin but your cells don't respond to it properly. Type II diabetes can often be reversed with lifestyle changes.

Gestational diabetes only occurs during pregnancy. It develops in the third trimester and doesn't usually cause any noticeable symptoms, so your partner will be tested for it at a prenatal visit between 24 and 28 weeks. It's believed that in gestational diabetes, hormones from the placenta keep the woman from producing as much insulin she needs or from being able to use the insulin she does produce.

The growing baby is the loser in this tug-of-war between insulin and blood sugar. Insulin doesn't cross the placenta but glucose does, putting the baby in danger of developing high blood sugar, or hyperglycemia, in the uterus. This can cause problems for the baby both before and after birth.

Gestational diabetes can usually be managed with exercise, a healthy diet and careful monitoring of blood sugar levels. Sometimes, though, a woman may temporarily need insulin.

Gestational diabetes should resolve once the baby is born, but there is a risk the woman will go on to develop Type II diabetes afterward. If your partner develops gestational diabetes, her blood sugar will be monitored after the baby comes to make sure it returns to normal.

## *Gestational hypertension*

Some women with normal blood pressure (120/80 or less) will develop high blood pressure (140/90 or higher) while pregnant, usually around 20 weeks. Sometimes it gets high enough to be worrisome, but it usually doesn't cause any problems and goes back to normal after the baby is born. It does increase the possibility the woman will develop chronic hypertension in the future, though.

## *Preeclampsia*

When a pregnant woman develops high blood pressure and signs of injury to vital organs like her kidneys or liver, this is called preeclampsia. Preeclampsia is very serious and has to be managed carefully to keep it from becoming life-threatening. Whereas gestational hypertension tends not to have any symptoms, preeclampsia can cause headaches, vision problems, abdominal pain, trouble breathing and swelling of the hands and face. Symptoms like these indicate preeclampsia is developing and urgent medical care is needed.

If your partner becomes preeclamptic she may be admitted to the hospital for treatment. The only cure for preeclampsia is to deliver the baby, so if she is at least 37 weeks along this will be strongly recommended. If she isn't yet at 37 weeks every effort will be made to keep her condition under control until she gets there, but if it can't be controlled the baby will need to be delivered anyway.

## *Problems with the placenta*

The two main problems that can develop with the placenta are called placenta previa and placenta abruption.

Until the baby is born and begins breathing on its own, it is completely dependent on the placenta for its oxygen. The placenta remains attached to the uterus throughout labor and birth, absorbing oxygen from mom's blood and passing it to the baby through the umbilical cord. If the placenta separates from the uterus before the baby is born, the effects can be catastrophic.

A Previa is when the placenta attaches very low in the uterus, partly or completely covering the cervix. Sometimes, as the baby grows and the uterus expands, the placenta will be pulled up away from the cervix. If this doesn't happen the baby will have to be delivered by cesarean section.

An abruption is when the placenta pulls away from the uterine wall before the baby is born. This can happen slowly or all at once. If it happens slowly over the course of the pregnancy the baby may be deprived of oxygen and nutrients. If it happens suddenly the baby can die. The heavy bleeding from a sudden abruption can be life-threatening for the mother as well.

## *Postdates/overdue*

When your partner first found out she was pregnant, her estimated due date (EDD) was calculated by adding 280 days to the first day of her last period. That works out to a little over nine months, or 40 weeks to be more exact. At each of her prenatal appointments and during any ultrasounds she has, the baby is measured, its state of development is determined and the EDD adjusted accordingly.

A full-term pregnancy has been defined in different ways through the years, but that 40-week standard has stuck. Generally, a baby born between about 39 and 41 weeks is considered full-term. Earlier than 39 weeks is early, and more than 41 weeks is late. These are just guidelines, however, as perfectly healthy babies may be born at 38 or 42 weeks.

If labor hasn't started by 42 weeks at the latest, though, medical intervention will be strongly advised. A baby who stays in the womb longer than this may grow so big it's hard to deliver. It may also suffer as the placenta starts to deteriorate and the number of amniotic fluid drops. There's also an increased risk of stillbirth.

You can be sure that by 40 weeks your partner will be done with being pregnant and will want very much for the baby to come. Some women find walking as much as possible helps. If the baby hasn't settled into a good position for birth it may be possible to use gravity and body movements to persuade it to do so. Certain herbal teas or extracts are sometimes suggested. Nipple stimulation and orgasm are often recommended to get the uterus contracting. Your partner should check in with her doctor or midwife before trying any of these.

## *Medical interventions to get labor started*

### *Ripening the cervix*

The primary measure of how well labor is progressing is the dilation and effacement, or opening and thinning, of the cervix. There are a number of different substances that can be applied directly to the cervix to "ripen" it, or cause it to soften. Sometimes ripening the cervix is enough to get labor started. Otherwise, it's done to prepare the cervix before induction, because the closer to ready the cervix is, the more likely induction will be successful.

## *Amniotomy*

The amniotic sac in which the baby floats in its amniotic fluid nearly always ruptures before birth, although rarely in a sudden, dramatic cascade as it does on TV. If your partner's cervix has thinned out and started to dilate and the baby's head is pressing on it—basically, at the starting gate, waiting for the race to begin—the doctor or midwife might go ahead and rupture the membranes. When the rupture is intentional it's called an amniotomy. In many cases, this will jump-start contractions and get labor going. Once the membranes have ruptured, though, whether naturally or through amniotomy, the clock starts ticking, as the baby is now unprotected from an infection that could reach it through the vagina. If amniotomy doesn't work to get labor started, the next step is induction or C-section.

## *Induction*

If your partner hasn't gone into labor naturally by 41 or 42 weeks, and if the baby looks healthy and like it will still fit through the birth canal, labor may be induced.

This is done in the hospital, by infusing Pitocin intravenously. Pitocin is a synthetic form of oxytocin, the hormone responsible for uterine contractions. It has a bad reputation for causing severely painful contractions but managed properly it can bring on contractions that slowly increase in intensity just like they naturally would.

The benefit of getting labor started with Pitocin has to be weighed against the risks, which include causing stress on the baby. If your partner has had a C-section previously, strong Pitocin contractions increase the risk of the uterus rupturing along the old incision. And not every Pitocin induction is successful; if labor still doesn't progress, a C-section could still be necessary.

# Chapter 11:
# Going into labor

So this is how it works: you and your partner are going about your normal business, maybe having a nice dinner, when suddenly she grabs her belly and gasps, "Honey, it's time!" Maybe her water breaks first, flooding the floor beneath her, and with wide eyes, she exclaims, "The baby is coming!" Then you jump in the car or taxi, possibly leaving her behind in your haste, and race to the hospital. Hopefully, you get there in time and she makes it to a bed before she starts sweating and screaming at the top of her lungs and the baby comes shooting out.

Right?

LOL. Forget everything you think you know about labor and childbirth from TV and movies. There is such a thing as precipitous labor that is short and sweet, but that's extremely rare. For most women, especially first-time moms, the reality is much, much different.

For one thing, her labor is very unlikely to start suddenly and obviously. The segue from Braxton Hicks "practice" contractions to "real" labor contractions can be very subtle. It may take hours or even days for your partner to be sure something different is going on. Even then, it probably isn't time to race off to the hospital.

Here's a quick timeline of the stages of labor. Later, we'll talk more about the actual birth.

## *Stages of labor*

The uterus is a muscular organ. In labor, the uterus contracts, pulling the cervix open and pushing the baby down and out. How long labor and each of its stages lasts is variable. For a first-time mom, there's usually at least 24 hours between the time she realizes she's in labor and the birth of the baby.

### *First stage*

The first stage of labor is when the cervix opens, or dilates, and thins out, or effaces. It's broken down into three phases of its own that are defined by what's going on with the cervix.

Phase one: Early labor

Phase one goes until the cervix has dilated 3 cm, roughly the size of a quarter. Some women will have already dilated to 1 cm weeks before labor starts. During this phase, contractions are noticeable but tend to be irregular and relatively mild. Your partner may feel like she has menstrual cramps, and she may feel the contractions in her back. They last about 30 to 45 seconds, anywhere from 5 to 30 minutes in between. It's hard to say how long this phase will take—it could be days. Your partner will stay in touch with her doctor or midwife during early labor but most likely will stay at home.

Phase two: Active labor

During active labor, the cervix dilates to 7 cm, about the diameter of a peach. Contractions get longer, stronger and closer together, lasting 45 to 60 seconds with about three to five minutes in between. If your partner is delivering at a hospital or birth center, this is the time to go there—safely, not in a panic. If you're having a home birth the midwife and doula or birth assistant will be in attendance.

### Phase three: Transition

This is the part where women on TV grab their partners by the collar and curse at them. As her cervix approaches 10 cm dilation, about the diameter of grapefruit, your partner could become quite emotional—don't take any outbursts personally. She may already be feeling the urge to push, but she'll have to fight that urge until the cervix is fully open. Starting to push before the cervix is ready can cause it to swell so that it not only stops opening, it actually closes some. You will have learned some techniques in your childbirth preparation classes to help her through this phase, so use them!

## *Second stage*

This is it! The second stage is when her cervix is fully dilated and your partner can begin pushing. As with the other stages, it's hard to say how long this one will last, but as with the others, it's usually longer for a first-time mom. Minutes or hours, this stage is hard work and can be grueling. With the finish line in sight your partner may be energized and determined, but if it takes a while she can become exhausted and discouraged. She will need your support now more than ever.

Once the baby is born it will be quickly examined to make sure there are no problems, the cord will be cut, and it will be placed on mom's chest so the three of you can start bonding and getting acquainted. However, if the baby needs any kind of special care it may be taken out of the room and the bonding will have to wait.

### *Third stage*

The delivery of the placenta is the least-glamorous stage of labor, but it still requires the careful attention of the doctor or midwife. They will examine the placenta carefully to make sure it's intact. Any pieces left behind can interfere with the uterus contracting back to its normal size, and that can cause serious bleeding. Fortunately, this is not at all common. It is more likely the placenta will be whole and everything will proceed normally.

When making your birth plan you and your partner probably discussed what, if anything, you wanted to do with the placenta. Some couples will take their home and use it to nourish a tree they plant in honor of their child's birth. There are those who advocate eating the placenta, something other mammals do, although there's no scientific basis for claims about its nutritional value. You and your partner may not really care what happens to the placenta, and that's fine, too. Leave it behind and it will be disposed of properly.

# Chapter 12:

# Who's going to be there when the baby comes?

Just as there are many ways to give birth, there are many kinds of healthcare practitioners who may be involved. Your individual cast of characters may end up including only those you know and expect, or there may stand-ins, understudies or unexpected walk-ons. It's good to know who might be there.

If you are having multiples or if there are other special circumstances, more specialties may be represented. Here are the ones most commonly involved in normal, uncomplicated deliveries.

## *Obstetrician*

An obstetrician, or OB, is a medical doctor who specializes in pregnancy and childbirth. A gynecologist, or GYN, specializes in women's reproductive health other than pregnancy and childbirth. An OB/GYN does both, and may even serve as a woman's primary care provider.

Doctors are generally trained to be in charge, and you can expect an OB to take a more directive approach to manage your partner's pregnancy. An OB is authorized to handle complications that arise during labor and delivery, including performing C-sections. In an uncomplicated vaginal delivery, the OB is often not present during labor and arrives just in time to "catch" the baby as it's born.

## *Certified nurse-midwife (CNM)*

A CNM is an advanced practice registered nurse who has post-graduate training in women's reproductive care and childbirth. You might think of a CNM as the nurse equivalent of an OB/GYN, but neither professional would be happy with that comparison. CNMs deliver babies in hospitals, birth centers and at home. Their scope of practice varies from state to state; in some places, they practice with a medical doctor and in some places there are independent. They may or may not be able to do forceps or vacuum deliveries, and while they may assist at C-sections they don't make the incision. CNMs tend to take a more collaborative approach to manage pregnancy and birth. Their focus is on uncomplicated pregnancy and delivery with minimal medical intervention.

## *Other kinds of midwives*

Some midwives enter the field by paths other than nursing. They are not nurses and don't do hospital deliveries, focusing instead on birth centers and home births. Certified midwives (CMs) complete post-graduate training on the same level as CNMs and take the same certification exam, although they are certified by a different professional board. Currently, only a few states license CMs. Certified professional midwives (CPMs) meet their educational and practice criteria through apprenticeships or through midwifery schools, but don't have post-graduate degrees. Their scope of practice depends on state law and is less comprehensive than that of CMs. They are currently licensed in most but not all states. Lay midwives typically have no formal training, certification or licensing.

## *Labor, delivery and postpartum nurses*

If your partner gives birth in a hospital, most of her care is likely to be provided by nurses who specialize in labor, delivery and postpartum care. These are the professionals who will be checking the fetal monitor and your partner's cervix, providing encouragement and nourishment and coordinating the rest of the care team. After the birth, they will weigh and measure the baby, poke its heel for blood tests and give vaccines. They'll monitor your partner's recovery and offer assistance with bathing, diapering, and breastfeeding.

## *Lactation consultant*

Babies and breasts are made to go together, but sometimes help is needed to get breastfeeding started. If your partner doesn't have friends or family members who have breastfed, she may just be unfamiliar with the process and need a little guidance. If she has inverted nipples, which point inward instead of outward, or if the baby has a cleft palate or other problem that interferes with feeding, a lactation consultant may be called in.

## *Birth assistant*

If you choose a birth center or home birth with a midwife, you may also have a birth assistant. Sometimes the birth assistant is hired by the midwife, and sometimes you hire the birth assistant directly with the midwife's approval. A birth assistant is a professional who has the background and training to assist the midwife; they may be a nurse, or they may have specific birth assistant certification. If for some reason you are transferred to a hospital for the birth, an assistant you have hired directly might come along and serve as a doula.

## *Doula*

A doula serves more as a companion and as a knowledgeable, supportive friend than a healthcare provider. She (doulas are overwhelmingly female) will not be involved in the medical or nursing aspects but will offer emotional and comfort care during pregnancy, labor, and childbirth. The difference between a doula and you, the woman's partner, is that the doula will have done this before, and may have experienced it all herself, first hand.

## *Anesthesiologist or nurse anesthetist*

If your partner opts for an epidural or other kind of numbing pain relief, this will be done by a medical doctor called an anesthesiologist or by an advanced practice nurse known as a nurse anesthetist. Once the epidural or other anesthesia is in place they will return to check it, but the moment-to-moment monitoring will be done by the labor and delivery nurses.

# Chapter 13:
# Childbirth methods and gear

Giving birth is the most natural thing in the world, but it isn't easy. It's hard work, it hurts and things don't always go according to plan. Your partner may want all the medical interventions, or she may want to try to manage without them. Here's a quick roundup of the approaches you can choose from, and some of the equipment you can expect to have on hand during the birth.

## *Lamaze*

The Lamaze method, developed by a French obstetrician of the same name, was introduced in the US in the 1950s. Originally focused on breathing techniques, a typical Lamaze course now covers 12 hours of instruction and aims to teach the woman and her partner a number of strategies for being active, effective participants in the birth process. Lamaze acknowledges that a woman may opt for pain control and that C-sections are sometimes necessary. As always, though, the goal is to minimize medical intervention.

## *Bradley*

The Bradley method, also known as "husband-coached childbirth," was devised by an

American obstetrician in the 1940s. Like Lamaze, it emphasizes that childbirth is a normal, natural process and encourages the woman and her partner to be active participants. The primary difference between Lamaze and Bradley is that while Lamaze offers ways to distract from the pain, Bradley teaches a relaxed acceptance of pain. The Bradley method also has a stronger emphasis on avoiding medical interventions.

### *Leboyer*

In the 1970s Leboyer, another French obstetrician introduced the radical notion that childbirth should take the baby's experience into account. He felt it was unnecessarily traumatic to pull a baby from its warm, cozy womb directly into a loud, cold, brightly-lit delivery room. As much as we may consider the baby's first cry as a triumphant confirmation of life, Leboyer saw it is a heartbreaking sign of the baby's distress. A Leboyer birth is quiet, dimly lit and, optimally, includes easing the baby into terrestrial life by delivering it into a warm bath, or placing it in a warm bath immediately after birth.

## *Water birth*

Before its birth, a baby spends its entire life floating in warm, nourishing fluid. Many consider a water birth to be the most natural way possible to ease a newborn into life outside the womb. This can also be deeply soothing and relaxing for the woman, especially if she feels a special affinity for water. Being delivered into water is considered safe for the baby because it usually won't try to breathe until it leaves the water and is exposed to air. A water birth usually takes place in an inflatable tub, much like a child's backyard pool, made for the purpose. Water birth is contraindicated in some situations, such as if the woman has genital herpes or the baby is breech or there are other possible complications.

## *Vaginal birth after cesarean (VBAC)*

It was once considered too risky for a woman to attempt a vaginal delivery if she had a previous C-section. It was thought the woman's uterus might rupture where it had been cut before. Years of study have shown this is uncommon and that most women who have had a C-section can safely give birth vaginally afterward. This will depend, of course, on why the previous section was done. Some hospitals still consider VBAC unacceptably risky and won't allow it to be attempted under any circumstances.

## Gear for labor and childbirth

### *Fetal monitor*

While the Doppler is great for doing a quick check on the baby's heart rate, more detailed information on how things are going is obtained with a fetal monitor, which also tracks the frequency and length of the woman's contractions. The most common kind of fetal monitor has two belts that wrap around the woman's belly, one for the baby's heart rate and one for contractions. If she has an epidural she'll stay in bed with the monitor on; otherwise, when she wants to get up and walk around, the monitor belts need to be taken off.

Less commonly, fetal monitoring may be done internally. With this method, a wired electrode is threaded through the woman's vagina and cervix and placed directly on the baby. Usually, the baby's head is the part that is most readily available, and that's where the electrode goes; it's actually screwed into the baby's scalp. Optionally, a device called an intrauterine pressure catheter can be inserted into the uterus to measure the force of uterine contractions. This kind of monitoring allows the woman to move around more than if she had an external monitor, but less than if she had no monitor at all. Internal monitoring may be more accurate than external monitoring, but it does have some risks. Infection is one concern, and internal monitoring can't be used if the mother has herpes, HIV or hepatitis.

## *Birthing ball*

A birthing ball, or birth ball, is just like the big exercise balls you use at the gym. Your partner can use one at home during pregnancy both as a comfortable place to sit and as a way to gently work the muscles in her back and abdomen. In labor, she may find it soothing to sit on the ball and bounce or rotate her pelvis in a circular motion. She can also put the ball either on the floor or on the bed and lean over it. It's possible to sit on the ball while in bed, but this can be tricky.

## *Peanut ball*

A peanut ball is a little like two smaller birth balls joined in the middle. It's used like a birthing ball but is more stable and safer to use while in bed. This is especially true when the woman has an epidural; there's some evidence that using a peanut ball with an epidural helps keep labor progressing and makes a C-section less likely.

### *Birthing bar*

A birthing bar, or squat bar, is a frame that can be attached to the end of a bed. The woman can hold onto the bar or drape her arms over it while squatting.

### *Birthing stool*

A birthing stool is a short stool that has the center cut out and an opening in the front, so that the seat is C-shaped. It takes the pressure off a woman's legs while she squats.

*Forceps*

There are different kinds of obstetrical forceps, but in general, they look something like salad tongs. They are used when the baby's head is within reach but has stopped moving down, if it's turned in a way that's making it hard for it to negotiate the birth canal, or if changes in its heart rate indicate delivery needs to be sped up. Once the forceps are in place, the doctor or midwife can apply steady pressure while the woman pushes, helping to ease the baby out. If necessary, they can turn the baby's head. Forceps are pretty safe, although they may leave some minor bruises on baby's head and an episiotomy may be needed.

*Vacuum extraction*

Also known as vacuum-assisted delivery, with vacuum extraction a suction cup is applied to the top of the baby's head and a vacuum pump used to help pull the baby out. It's used for the same kind of reasons as forceps.

# Chapter 14:
# Complications in labor and childbirth

## *Preterm labor and premature birth*

Labor that starts before the $37^{th}$ week of pregnancy is called preterm labor, and a baby born this early is considered premature. In the past premature babies often didn't survive, but nowadays it isn't unusual for babies born at 25 weeks (and sometimes even earlier) to make it. The more premature a baby is, of course, the more medical care will be needed to help it mature enough to leave the hospital.

Sometimes Braxton Hicks contractions become increasingly intense in the last trimester and can be confused with preterm labor. Braxton Hicks contractions cause a generalized tightening of uterine muscles and some discomfort similar to mild menstrual cramps, but they don't cause the cervix to open. True labor contractions get increasingly painful, longer-lasting and closer together. It's never wrong to check in with your partner's doctor or midwife if she isn't sure what kind of contractions she's having.

## *Cervical incompetence*

Also called cervical insufficiency or an incompetent cervix, this is when the cervix begins to thin and open too early in pregnancy, risking miscarriage or premature delivery. Cervical incompetence isn't common. Some known or suspected risk factors include certain genetic disorders and having had a previous dilation and curettage (a procedure where the cervix is opened so the uterus can be accessed). Often there's no known risk factor.

Cervical incompetence typically doesn't cause any symptoms in the first trimester, but in the second trimester may feel a little like early labor, with pressure in the pelvis and vaginal spotting. If your partner is diagnosed with an incompetent cervix, various treatments may be tried to prevent premature labor or loss of the pregnancy. The most invasive treatment is called cervical cerclage, in which the cervix is actually sutured shut. The sutures are removed near the due date or when labor begins.

## *Premature rupture of membranes (PROM)*

A baby in the uterus floats in amniotic fluid, which is enclosed in the amniotic sac. The amount of amniotic fluid within the membranes increases until about 34 weeks, when there may be as much as 800 ml (about 27 ounces, or almost three-and-a-half cups). After that it starts to drop, until by 40 weeks there are about 600 ml of fluid.

The event popularly known as the woman's water breaking is the amniotic sac, or membranes, rupturing so the amniotic fluid escapes. This normally happens during labor, although in very rare cases babies are born with the membranes intact. PROM happens before labor starts, sometimes well before. The amniotic fluid may all empty at once, as it does on TV, or it may leak out slowly.

The pregnancy may be able to continue with a slow leak, as amniotic fluid is continually replaced, but the baby can't survive in the uterus without any fluid at all. When a great deal of fluid is lost through PROM, the baby will have to be delivered. If labor doesn't begin naturally, either it will be induced or the baby will be delivered by cesarean section.

## *Shoulder dystocia*

Dystocia means difficult childbirth, and shoulder dystocia is when the birth is complicated by the baby's shoulders not fitting through the birth canal. Sometimes ultrasounds will offer an advance warning of potential shoulder dystocia, and a cesarean section will probably be scheduled. Sometimes, though, the problem is unexpected and only becomes obvious after the baby's head is already out.

It might seem obvious that very big babies would be most likely to have shoulder dystocia, but most big babies don't have it, and most babies who do have it aren't exceptionally large. When shoulder dystocia does occur, the doctor or midwife will try a range of workarounds that may include changing the woman's position, performing an episiotomy, or manipulating the baby by reaching into the birth canal or pressing on it through the woman's abdomen. Fortunately, these maneuvers are usually successful.

## *Meconium aspiration*

Even though a baby in the womb gets its nutrition through the placenta, by the second trimester it will begin swallowing amniotic fluid. Some of the fluid will be recycled as urine, which is part of why the volume of amniotic fluid increases. Amniotic fluid contains more than just water, though; in addition to the discarded skin cells that make amniocentesis possible, there may be lanugo, or fetal hair, and other bits and pieces. This organic matter accumulates in the baby's gut and forms its first poop, which is called meconium.

Normally meconium makes its appearance in the newborn's first few diapers, but sometimes it finds its way into the amniotic fluid before birth. This usually happens when the baby becomes distressed during labor, but sometimes there isn't any obvious reason for it.

If the baby swallows meconium, it can be pulled into the airway when it takes its first breaths. Often suctioning the airways is enough to keep problems from developing, but if the meconium makes its way down into the baby's lungs the baby may need to be admitted to the hospital for medical care.

## *Stalled labor*

Labor is hard work, and at times your partner might wish it would stop. What she never wants before the baby comes, though, is for it to actually stop. Stalled labor is when contractions slow or stop altogether, or when they continue but without opening the cervix. This can be discouraging and exhausting and increases the risk of ending up with a C-section.

Although the idea is outdated, many healthcare providers still believe that once a woman is in active labor, her cervix should open by at least 1 cm per hour. A midwife in a birth center or home birth may be willing to let slow labor take its course (as long as mom and baby are okay), but in a hospital, it will only be tolerated for so long before intervention is recommended.

It's important that you and your partner talk about your commitment to vaginal delivery and make this clear in your birth plan. Recognize, of course, that things may not go as wished or planned, and that your feelings may change once things are underway. But decide ahead of time what kind of approach you want to take if labor stalls. Do you want to accept recommended medical interventions to keep things going? Or do you want to do whatever you can to avoid intervention?

What needs to be done to get stalled labor going again depends on what's causing it to slow.

## *What you and your partner can do*

### Change position

Sometimes labor slows because the baby isn't in that ideal head-down, facing mom's spine position. She may be able to use a combination of gravity, walking and body movements to persuade the baby to settle into a better position. Even if she's in bed with an epidural, it's possible to help her move around. Your midwife, doula, nurse or birth assistant will be able to suggest safe, effective movements and positions.

## Nipple stimulation

Rubbing or kneading your partner's nipples may cause a release of oxytocin, a hormone that acts on the uterus. (In fact, if she was in danger of preterm labor she may have been told to avoid nipple stimulation for this reason.) This is something either you or she can do. Another good way for her to boost oxytocin release is to have an orgasm; this is something you might have tried at home if the baby was overdue and you wanted to get labor started. It's the rare woman who will be enthusiastic about this option while in labor—especially if she's in the hospital—but it might be worth consideration.

Check with the midwife or nurse to make sure it's safe to try this option.

Take a shower

A warm shower can be very relaxing, and letting the water run over her breasts may provide some gentle nipple stimulation to get that oxytocin flowing.

## *What healthcare providers can do*

If you are having a birth center or home birth, the midwife will help you with strategies to get a stalled labor going again naturally. If you are in a hospital, the go-to intervention is Pitocin or augmented labor. Pitocin is a synthetic form of oxytocin that's infused intravenously. The advantage of Pitocin is that it's very effective at stimulating contractions. The disadvantage is that it can cause contractions that go from zero to excruciating in a very short time, sometimes leading to fetal distress or the need for labor-slowing pain relief. It's possible, though, for a carefully managed Pitocin infusion to mimic natural contractions.

# Chapter 15:
# The birth itself

Back in the day, the laboring woman was whisked off to a private area and her partner was directed to the waiting room, where he paced and fretted, clutching a fistful of cigars, anxiously wondering if everything was okay. Eventually, a doctor or nurse arrived at the door to inform him of the arrival of his son or daughter (surprise!) and invite him to visit his family.

Nowadays it's pretty much assumed you're going to be there to support your partner during labor, to witness the birth of your child and perhaps to have a hand in the proceedings. If you think pregnancy was a mental and emotional rollercoaster, wait until you experience childbirth!

## *Labor*

If everything you know about having babies comes from watching TV, you're in for a few surprises. A half-hour sitcom has to compress the entire process into just a few minutes, and it's much funnier when everything happens in a panicky rush. In reality, especially if this is your partner's first baby, you should expect least 24 hours to pass between the time your partner knows she's in labor to the sound of your baby's first cry. In fact, the earliest stage of labor, the part before you leave for the hospital or birth center or before the midwife arrives at your home, can take days.

*It takes time*

You may feel nervous and excited when labor begins, especially if you think it's going to be fast. After all the months of anticipation, it's go time! Then, as the hours go by, you may become worried, tired or even bored. If your partner has a doula or has asked another close friend or family member to be present, you may be able to take short breaks. Get something to eat, check your email, go for a walk (a short one!), catch your breath—then get back in there and support your partner.

*Epidurals can be weird*

If she has chosen to have an epidural, your partner may enter a kind of surreal situation where she sits comfortably in bed watching TV and playing cards, just as if it were any normal day. She'll have a fetal monitor strapped around her belly and the nurses will come in and look at the monitor to see how her contractions are going because she won't be feeling them. You may be either relieved or bewildered by this turn of events. It can almost feel like you're literally waiting for a delivery—like someone else is getting the baby ready and you're just waiting for them to show up.

Otherwise, as your partner progresses through the stages of labor you can expect the action to get more intense and your attention (and hers!) to become much more focused. You might have been able to pop out for short breaks early on, but as she gets closer to pushing, and absolutely while she's pushing, you'll have to be fully present.

### *Push!*

Once your partner's cervix is fully dilated and ready to let the baby through, she will finally be given the go-ahead to start pushing. This is likely to be a huge relief for her, as the urge to push can be overwhelming and she may have been fighting it up to that moment. She'll push during her contractions, which will by now be long and close together. This is very hard work! She may push for anywhere from a few minutes to a couple of hours. The baby's heart rate will be checked frequently and she can push as long as she needs to, provided she has the energy and the baby is okay. If she starts to tire, the baby isn't moving down or its heart rate indicates distress, possible interventions to speed up the delivery include episiotomy, forceps and vacuum extraction.

## *Crowning*

At some point a doctor, midwife or nurse is likely to announce the baby is crowning, meaning the top of its head is clearly visible. This is an exciting development because the rest of the baby isn't far behind and birth is imminent. Depending on where you are, a mirror may be set up so your partner can see the baby's head crowning. This shows her that all is well and she's nearly done, which may be all the incentive she needs to power through the last few contractions.

If you are at the head of the bed with her or supporting her from behind, you can watch in the mirror, too. If you are holding her hand but she doesn't want you any closer than that, you might find yourself looking directly at the emerging baby.

Either way, there's a lot to take in, and a lot of ways to feel about it. At this point, your partner's vagina will not look anything like its usual self. It may be hard to believe it was once so inviting, or that it ever will be again. There will be stretching, and possibly tearing, and likely some bleeding. Pushing a small human being through the vagina also puts quite a strain on the neighboring rectum. If your partner didn't have visible hemorrhoids before, she might now. In fact, the inside of her rectum itself may put in an appearance. Many women poop a little while pushing. None of these things are unexpected and all become irrelevant once the baby comes.

## *Cesarean section*

If your baby is delivered by cesarean, things will go a little differently. Your partner may have tried to deliver vaginally and ended up with an unexpected C-section, or it may have been planned in advance for various reasons. Either way, it will take place in a surgical suite. If your partner already has an epidural in place, it will provide the numbing she needs for the operation. Otherwise, an epidural or another kind of numbing procedure will be used to make her comfortable. In very rare cases, if an epidural is not in place and the C-section is extremely urgent, general anesthesia may be used.

You will usually be allowed to stay with your partner for the C-section. It's still surgery, though, so you'll change into scrubs and may wear a surgical mask to wear over your nose and mouth or a cap to cover your hair. You'll be able to talk to and reassure your partner, and you'll await your baby's arrival together. As with vaginal delivery, if the baby checks out okay it will be placed on mom's chest where you'll start getting acquainted while her incision is sutured.

## *The newborn*

You may find your newborn baby to be the most miraculously beautiful thing you've ever seen, and fall head over heels in love at first sight. Or, you may find he or she looks like a gooey little extraterrestrial, and wonder how you will ever love him or her. Either reaction, or anything in between, is perfectly normal. Don't judge yourself if your feelings aren't immediately positive; sometimes the love grows slowly. But do keep any negative reactions to yourself. They might make for a funny story someday, but your partner doesn't want to hear it right now.

Some newborns are plump, clear-skinned and Instagram-ready. Some have red skin, angry faces, and cone-shaped heads. They may be covered in a creamy biofilm called vernix, or lanugo, a kind of soft hair all over the body. If forceps or vacuum extraction were used, the head or face may be bruised. Again, all perfectly normal and not at all predictive of they will look like in the days to come.

A newborn is typically most alert in the first hour or two after birth. Your baby may yawn, squirm, grasp your finger, look at your face and recognize your voice. Your partner won't be making milk yet but will be encouraged to put the baby to her breast, which the baby should willingly do. Enjoy this time, because soon he or she will fall asleep and it may be a while before you get to interact like this again.

### *Assessing the newborn*

The doctor or midwife attending the birth will be less concerned with your baby's good looks than with whether he or she looks good, health-wise. They will use the Apgar score to quickly determine if the baby has any problems that need addressing.

You may read that Apgar stands for "Appearance, Pulse, Grimace, Activity and Respiration," but that's just a memory aid. It's actually named after Virginia Apgar, the American doctor who invented it. An Apgar score is usually done at one minute and five minutes after delivery. The baby is given a score of 0, 1 or 2 on each of five criteria: heart rate, respiratory effort, muscle tone, reflexes, and color. A score of 7 to 10 indicates a healthy baby who needs just routine care. A lower score indicates continued monitoring is appropriate, and a very low or dropping score may mean it's time for medical intervention.

*Cutting the cord*

The umbilical cord, the baby's lifeline up until birth, is no longer needed once the baby is breathing air. The cord contains two arteries that carried oxygen-rich blood and nutrients to the baby in the uterus and one vein that carried depleted blood and waste away. Immediately after birth some transfer is still taking place, and you may notice the cord pulsing in time with your partner's heartbeat. As long as neither mom nor baby needs emergency care, there will be no rush to cut the cord; many midwives, especially, advocate for waiting for the pulsing to stop before cutting. Then they will put two clamps on the umbilical cord, cut in between the clamps, and place the baby on mom's chest. If you or your partner want to cut the cord, you'll be handed the scissors to do so. You may be surprised at how tough and gristle-like the cord is, so be ready. Not everyone wants to cut the cord; if you don't want to, just say no.

## *Cord blood*

Cord blood is the blood that remains in the placenta and the umbilical cord after the cord has been cut. It contains red and white blood cells, but it also contains the kind of blood-forming stem cells found in bone marrow. These stem cells, which can be used to treat a variety of life-threatening conditions, can be frozen and stored indefinitely. You can choose to donate your child's cord blood in the hopes it will be a good match for someone desperate for this kind of treatment, or you can pay to have it stored in case your family needs it in the future.

## *Breastfeeding*

If your partner plans to breastfeed, she will be encouraged to start right away. She won't have milk yet—nor will the baby need it yet—but the oxytocin released when the baby latches on to her breast will stimulate her uterus to contract to its non-pregnant size. This is critically important to prevent excessive bleeding. The oxytocin and physical closeness also help promote bonding.

## *The uterus*

You may notice the doctor, midwife or nurse pressing on your partner's belly after the baby and placenta have both been delivered. They are feeling her uterus to make sure it's firm, so the blood vessels that were attached to the placenta are compressed. If the uterus doesn't clamp down on the blood vessels they can bleed heavily. If the uterus feels too soft, they may massage it by pressing on your partner's abdomen. If this isn't enough, the doctor or midwife may massage the uterus with one hand on the abdomen and one in the vagina. Pitocin, the synthetic oxytocin analog, may also be given. In the very unlikely case, your partner's uterus doesn't respond to these measures, surgery may be needed.

## *Episiotomy and perineal tears*

You have probably wondered from time to time how it's even possible for a 7- or 8-pound baby to pass through your partner's vagina. No doubt your partner has spent some time thinking about this as well! What kind of magic makes it possible for her to pass a baby-size package through that small space?

Nature takes care of all of this, softening and loosening ligaments in the pelvis and lending elasticity to vaginal tissues so they can stretch and then return (or nearly return) to their pre-baby size. But skin and muscle can only stretch so far, and sometimes a baby needs a bit more space than mom's vagina can accommodate. Something has to give, and that something is her perineum.

The perineum is the space between the vagina and the anus. Sometimes the perineum will tear during childbirth, and sometimes the doctor or midwife will cut it. The cut is called an episiotomy. Healthcare practitioners may have strong opinions as to whether cutting or tearing is better. There are advantages and disadvantages to each.

Perineal tears may be minor or major. There are four degrees of tearing, depending on how many layers of tissue are involved and how far toward the rectum they go. One advantage of letting the perineum tear is that the least severe tear, which doesn't extend all the way to the muscle, is easier to repair and recover from than a cut that goes all the way through. The major disadvantage of letting the perineum tear is that the doctor or midwife has no control over how severe the tear turns out to be. A full-thickness tear that reaches into the rectum can be a life-changing injury for the woman.

The main advantage of an episiotomy is that the doctor or midwife controls how far the cut goes. The main disadvantage is that the cut goes all the way through connective tissue and muscle and so may be more painful and take longer to heal than a superficial tear. There was a time when episiotomies were routine and nearly always done, but this is no longer the case.

If your partner has a perineal tear or episiotomy, some special care will be needed. A first-degree tear doesn't usually need to be repaired, but an episiotomy or a more severe tear will need to be sutured. If she doesn't have an epidural in place she'll be given a local anesthetic to numb the area while the suturing is done. Afterward, she'll be given a squirt bottle for cleaning and will need to monitor for signs of infection or other complications, just as she would for any other kind of incision or injury.

Even without tearing or cutting, your partner's perineum is likely to feel sore and a little fragile after a vaginal delivery. Childbirth is normal and natural, but that doesn't mean it's easy! When it's time to have a bowel movement she may feel like "everything is going to fall out" if she does any pushing. Applying counter-pressure to the perineum with a pad of toilet paper or gauze will help with this.

# Chapter 16:
# Cesarean section

As a rule, the female body is well-adapted to the task of delivering a baby through the birth canal, in what we call a vaginal delivery. The human species wouldn't have lasted as long as it has if procreation couldn't proceed naturally and without medical help.

That being said, vaginal delivery is sometimes not advisable and sometimes simply not possible. In these cases, the baby is delivered through cesarean section, commonly known as a C-section. In a C-section, an incision is made through the woman's abdomen and into the uterus, and the baby is delivered through the incision. This is easier on mom and baby in some ways but has its drawbacks as well.

Sometimes a C-section is planned and is scheduled for a particular date and time. The obvious advantage for you and your partner is that you know exactly when the baby is coming. Sometimes a vaginal delivery is planned but something occurs during labor that makes a C-section necessary. This may be worrisome or disappointing, but the aim is to ensure a healthy mom and baby.

## *Reasons for planned C-section*

*Breech or transverse baby*

Late in pregnancy but before labor starts the baby usually "drops," or settles into position for birth. The ideal position is head down, facing mom's spine. A baby who settles with feet or butt down is called breech. Breech babies can be delivered vaginally, and many have been, but there are risks involved and nowadays many practitioners cannot or will not attempt them.

Some hospitals don't allow vaginal breech deliveries, and in some places, breech births are considered high-risk and therefore outside the scope of a midwife's practice. A big concern is that in a breech birth the baby's head is delivered last, and unforeseen problems getting the head or shoulders through the birth canal could be disastrous.

A transverse baby is laying sideways, and obviously can't enter the birth canal like that. If efforts to persuade a transverse baby to turn are unsuccessful, a C-section will be necessary.

## *Genital herpes*

Herpes may be an uncomfortable inconvenience for you and your partner, but for a newborn baby it can cause devastating neurological damage or even death. If your partner has contracted herpes late in pregnancy she won't have any antibodies to pass on to the baby, putting the baby at risk of infection it can't fight off. If she contracted herpes well before this pregnancy her antibodies will help protect the baby. Nevertheless, if your partner has an active herpes outbreak as her due date approaches, a C-section will probably be recommended.

### *Mom's health problems*

Some medical conditions can make vaginal delivery dangerous for a woman. These include heart and brain conditions that may be aggravated by the strain of pushing and sometimes chronic or pregnancy-related conditions like diabetes or high blood pressure.

### *Obstructions*

In placenta previa, the placenta has attached low in the uterus and completely or partially blocks the cervix. Fibroids, which are noncancerous growths that can develop in the uterus, can also obstruct the cervix. Sometimes there is an obvious mismatch between the size of the baby's head or shoulders and the mother's pelvic opening.

## *Previous C-section*

If your partner has had a C-section before, she may be advised to have another one this time. It may be that the problem that led to the last C-section is still a problem. Also, there is a risk that during labor the uterus could rupture along the old incision, although this is less common with the way C-sections are done today.

A vaginal delivery after a C-section is called VBAC (vaginal birth after cesarean) and may or may not be advisable, depending on what kind of incision she had, how well she recovered and why it was done. About 60 percent to 80 percent of attempted VBACs are successful and result in safe vaginal delivery, but some hospitals will not allow them anyway.

### *Multiple births*

Sometimes twins are delivered vaginally if it looks like the delivery will be uncomplicated. If the position of one or both babies is problematic, a C-section may be scheduled for safety reasons. Triplets (or more!) are likely to be delivered by C-section because it's complicated to ensure the wellbeing of this many babies during labor and delivery.

## *Reasons for unplanned C-sections*

### *Fetal distress*

If during pregnancy your partner notices the baby is not moving as much as usual, her doctor or midwife will check the baby's heart rate and possibly do an ultrasound. If these aren't reassuring a C-section may be advised. If the baby shows signs of distress during labor, such as a heart rate that is too fast, too slow or irregular, an emergency C-section may be done.

### *Pre-eclampsia*

Pre-eclampsia, in which the woman develops high blood pressure and possible organ damage, that develops in the last trimester can sometimes reach crisis proportions as labor begins. The only definitive treatment for pre-eclampsia is to deliver the baby, so if it looks like it is progressing toward life-threatening eclampsia an emergency C-section will be done.

### *Labor is not progressing*

An important reason not to rush to the hospital at the first sign of labor is that the clock starts ticking the minute your partner is admitted.

At home or in a birth center a woman may be allowed to labor for days, but in a hospital, there's an expectation that labor will progress along a fairly standard timeline. Otherwise, interventions to speed things along will be suggested, sometimes firmly.

If these are not successful, or if hours of intense contractions are simply not opening the cervix, at some point a C-section becomes inevitable. This is especially true if your partner's water has broken early on; this is known as premature rupture of membranes, or PROM, and presents a risk of infection if the baby isn't born in a timely manner.

## *Umbilical prolapse*

This is when the umbilical cord, which the baby relies on for its oxygen, drops down into or through the cervix ahead of the baby. This can happen during labor but can also happen before labor begins, especially after PROM. Prolapse can cause compression of the umbilical cord, cutting off oxygen delivery to the baby. Depending on when it happens and how severe its effect on the baby, a C-section may be urgently needed.

# Chapter 17: Complications after delivery

## *Uterine atony*

Atony is a lack of muscle tone. The uterus is a muscular organ, and sometimes the way it is stretched and fatigued in pregnancy and childbirth can leave it lax and unresponsive. If this happens, the blood vessels where the placenta was attached to the lining of the uterus may continue to bleed. Your partner's uterus will be checked for firmness as soon as the placenta has been delivered. Normally it will be fine, and if it isn't a little massage is usually enough to get it started, but sometimes Pitocin is used. Some hospitals nowadays routinely give Pitocin to prevent atony.

## *Hemorrhage*

Your partner will have bleeding after giving birth, regardless of whether she had a vaginal delivery or a C-section. This normal postpartum shedding of blood and tissue, called lochia, continues as the uterus contracts back down to its non-pregnant size and the cervix closes. It may be fairly heavy at first, with noticeable clots. The blood may pool up in her vagina when she's resting and come out all at once when she stands up. The bleeding should gradually get lighter until it stops altogether, which may take several weeks. Because the cervix is still partially open, putting anything in the vagina during this time risks introducing infection into the uterus, so tampons and intercourse are no-noes.

If for any reason your partner's uterus is slow to contract, she may have excessive bleeding or hemorrhaging. Hemorrhage will be suspected if she has bright red blood for more than three days, if she passes very large clots or if she has symptoms of severe blood loss like feeling dizzy and clammy. It isn't very likely this will happen to your partner, but symptoms like these require medical follow up right away.

# Chapter 18:

# Now you have a baby!

## *Newborn care in the hospital/birth center*

If your baby is delivered in a hospital or birth center, the staff will have a few more tasks to perform while you and your partner celebrate and congratulate yourselves on a job well done.

### *Heel stick test*

At some point, a nurse will want to poke your baby's heel with a small lancet and squeeze out a few drops of blood onto a card. This card will then be sent off to a lab that will test for up to

30 different genetic conditions. The exact number of conditions tested for varies from state to state, but they all include certain conditions it's important to know about right away, like phenylketonuria (PKU). PKU is an inherited disorder that requires dietary treatment to prevent severe health problems. Another condition that is tested for, galactosemia, can potentially make breastfeeding dangerous for the baby, so it's important to know about it as soon as possible.

## *Weight and measurement*

If your partner got regular prenatal care, and especially if she had any late ultrasounds, the measurements done after your baby is born will pretty much confirm what was already known.

Your baby's length will be measured in inches; average length is 19 to 20 inches, although the normal range is more like 18 to 22 inches. The average weight is considered to be about 7.5 pounds, although anything from about 5.5 pounds to 10 pounds is considered normal. A newborn will usually lose a little water weight in the first few days, then start gaining again after that.

## *Hepatitis B vaccine*

Newborns are routinely given a first hepatitis B vaccine, with two more to follow in the coming months. Hepatitis B is a virus that attacks the liver. An infant or young child who is infected with hepatitis B is at risk of becoming seriously ill and developing liver failure or cancer. If your partner has hepatitis B she can pass the virus on to the baby. In this case, the baby will also need a dose of immune globulin to help fight off the infection.

As with other recommended vaccines you have the option of refusing this one. Just know that you don't have to be sexually active or a drug user to contract hepatitis B—the virus shows up in many people with no known risk factors, including children, and it can be transmitted by people who don't even know they have it. If you think you might refuse or postpone the hepatitis B vaccine, it's vitally important for your partner to be tested for it.

*Vitamin K*

Vitamin K, which is needed for blood clotting, doesn't cross the placenta very well and babies tend to be born without enough to protect them from excessive bleeding. They are at risk of vitamin K deficiency until they start eating solid food, usually around six months. An injection of vitamin K is recommended for every newborn to prevent bleeding during these first few months. Vitamin K can be given orally but it's less effective and requires repeated dosing. Breastmilk, while ideal for infant nutrition in nearly every way, doesn't contain much vitamin K. Infant formulas have vitamin K added but may not be sufficient if for any reason the baby doesn't get enough.

### *Erythromycin ointment*

The practice of putting erythromycin ointment in the eyes of newborn babies became nearly universal once it was realized it could seriously prevent eye infections in the first month of life. There are many agents of infection that can affect a baby's eyes, but the most serious are gonorrhea and chlamydia. All hospitals in the US will recommend the ointment, and in some states, it's mandated by law. Some other countries have dropped the requirement in favor of screening pregnant women for sexually transmitted infections (STIs). There are many reasons to be checked for STIs in pregnancy, and this is another reason why prenatal care is so important.

## *Footprints, fingerprints and identity bands*

Your baby may stay with you in your hospital room every minute from birth to discharge home, but you are likely to have at least a short times apart. To be sure the right baby goes home with the right mom, the baby's footprints and mom's fingerprints are taken. Traditionally the prints have been done with ink on paper, but some places are introducing electronic scanners that take digital prints instead. Mom, baby, and dad will be given matching ID bands to wear as well. Some hospitals place an electronic band on the baby's leg that will lock all the doors in the unit if the baby is taken too close to one of them. Any time a healthcare provider takes your baby out of your room, they should check ID bands when they come back. If they don't, speak up and remind them.

*Bathing*

Newborns can be a little messy right after they're born—they are dried off right away to keep them from getting chilled, but bits of blood and vernix, a creamy biofilm that forms on the skin in the womb, can stick to skin and hair. Hospital staff may offer to take your baby to the nursery for a bath or can help you do the bathing in your room. You may also choose *not* to bathe your baby yet. Any vernix that remains can be rubbed in instead of washed off, as it forms a protective barrier on the skin.

## More newborn care

*Umbilical stump*

After the umbilical cord is cut a portion of it, called the stump, remains attached to the baby.

At first, there will still be a plastic clamp on the stump, which will make it especially awkward. The clamp is to prevent bleeding through the stump until its blood vessels shut down completely. Once the cord is dry the clamp can be removed, generally within the first day or so. The stump, however, will remain for another two or three weeks, slowly shrinking and shriveling until it finally falls off, leaving behind your baby's cute little belly button. You'll have to keep the stump clean, diaper around it and watch for signs of infection. Fortunately, infection is uncommon; unfortunately, oozing of stinky goo is not. You and your partner will be given instructions on how to tell the difference between normal decay of this formerly living tissue and infection that needs treatment.

## *Jaundice*

Jaundice is a yellowing of the skin, and sometimes of the eyes, that is caused by a buildup of bilirubin. Bilirubin is a component of red blood cells that is released when old cells are broken down to make way for new ones, a process that goes on continuously in all of us. In the uterus, the baby's bilirubin is cleared through the placenta. After birth, the baby's liver needs to take over this function, but there can be a delay before it reaches full capacity. During this time even healthy full-term babies can become mildly jaundiced. Usually keeping the baby well-fed and spending some time in sunlight, even next to a window, is sufficient. More significant jaundice may require treatment with special lights, and in some cases with IV fluids. In rare cases, severe jaundice signals serious medical conditions that require aggressive medical management. You'll be given lots of information on how to monitor your baby for jaundice.

## *Circumcision and the foreskin*

Certainly, you and your partner will have discussed whether or not you want your son to be circumcised, and hopefully, you were in agreement! There was a time when male circumcision, whether just after birth or later, routine or ceremonial, was nearly universal in the US, but now many parents are choosing to forgo it. There are health, hygiene, and cosmetic considerations as well as religious and family traditions to weigh, but in the end, the choice is up to you. If you decide against circumcision, you'll need to learn about caring for your son's penis and foreskin. At birth, the foreskin will be attached to the glans, or head of the penis. In the time it will separate and can be retracted, but this could take anywhere from hours to years. Until then it should never be forcefully retracted, and you should only "clean what is seen." If you decide to go ahead with circumcision it can be done before you leave the hospital or, if your son was born outside a hospital, in the pediatrician's office. This is a relatively minor procedure but will require some aftercare to keep your son comfortable and prevent infection. If you have your son circumcised by a mohel, oral suction to remove the foreskin is strongly discouraged as it can transmit infection.

## *Going home*

The day has finally come! This is an exciting time for your new family! If you had your baby in a hospital, how long you stay before going home depends on whether your partner had a vaginal delivery or a C-section, and how well she and the baby are doing. If all is well and there are no complications, you can expect to head home in a day or two after a vaginal delivery and three or four days after a C-section.

*Car seat*

You'll be expected to provide a safe, properly fitting infant car seat the ride home, so don't forget it! Make sure you've practiced putting it in and taking it out of the car so you don't have to figure it out in real time.

## *Visitors*

The arrival of a new baby is an exciting time, and your friends and family will want to drop by to check out the newcomer and wish you well. There will be plenty of time for this, though, and it doesn't have to happen all at once. If you've been on an adrenaline high since the baby was born, you can be sure the crash is coming. All three of you need rest and nourishment. There is usually a bit of a honeymoon period when a newborn baby sleeps a lot and cries very little, and you will begin to think you have been blessed with the happiest, most chill kid ever. That isn't going to last, though, so sleep while you can.

You'll want to limit the number of visitors you have each day, how long they stay and the number that is present at one time. If they don't offer to bring food, wash dishes or run a load of laundry, ask them to do so. Anyone you can't be this direct with can wait to visit until you and your new family are more settled and can accommodate them.

Be ready to gently refuse entry to anyone who has a cold or any other contagious illness, no matter how minor. Yes, your baby will need exposure to germs to build a healthy immune system, but that's for later when his or her immune system has kicked in. Ask any visitor, even family, who wants to hold your baby to wash their hands first. Don't forget to stock up on hand sanitizer! And kissing is definitely out; as much as visitors may want to smooch those chubby little cheeks, exposure to the herpes virus at this age can be disastrous.

# Chapter 19:
# Baby care at home

At last, you're home. Visitors have departed, the house is quiet, and it's just you, your partner, and your new baby. Suddenly, it hits you: you've never done this before. What happens next? You've read all the books, watched all the videos and listened while friends and family gave you their best advice. But now that it's all real, you may feel a little overwhelmed.

Don't worry.

Whether you're on top of the world or scared to death, what you're feeling is perfectly normal. Sure, this is the most important project you'll ever take on. But you've got lots of time to figure things out and grow into the role. You'll get some things wrong, but you'll get many things right. Just be patient with yourself and your new little family. You got this.

## *Caring for your newborn*

Basically, newborn babies eat, sleep and poop. Oh, and cry. That's pretty much it. Let's look at each of those.

### *Eating*

Breastfeeding

Whatever other purposes they serve before and after, with a baby in the house breasts are for milk. Not every woman will breastfeed, of course; your partner may have reasons not to, and fortunately there are alternatives. But if she does, this will bring its own set of advantages and challenges.

The advantages are many. Breastfeeding:

- Meets baby's nutritional needs perfectly
- Leads to very mild-smelling baby poop
- Releases oxytocin, encouraging mother-baby bonding
- Stimulates mom's uterus to contract and return to non-pregnant size
- Lowers mom's risk of breast and uterine cancers
- Is super convenient!

There may be challenges, as well. Breastfeeding:

- Is natural but doesn't always feel natural at first

- Can be uncomfortable when nipples are tender or when breasts are engorged
- Requires mom to pump if she needs to be away from the baby
- Can feel awkward or even be discouraged in public places
- Limits what mom can wear, as breasts need to always be accessible
- Can make dad feel left out

Bottle feeding

Bottles make it possible for the baby to be fed if your partner needs to return to work or otherwise needs to be away, or if she isn't breastfeeding. A lot of research has gone into designing bottle nipples that babies find acceptable, and you may need to try a couple of different ones. Whether breastmilk or formula is in the bottle, being able to hold and feed your baby can help you enjoy the kind of bonding you might otherwise miss out on.

*Sleeping*

Immediately after birth your baby will probably have an hour or two of quiet alertness, then fall asleep. Every newborn is unique, of course, but many will then go on to stay relaxed and sleep pretty much full-time for the next couple of weeks. Then, for the next few months, a baby sleeps about 17 out of every 24 hours. They usually wake up hungry every three or four hours but breastfed babies often nurse for comfort, too, and may wake up wanting the breast even more often.

You may be tempted to tiptoe around, whispering and keeping the house perfectly quiet while your baby is sleeping, but this isn't necessary. First of all, there's a reason we use the expression "sleep like a baby." They're pretty good at it. Babies need to sleep, and yours will adapt to the ambient sound level. Better to live your normal life—within reason, of course. Excessive noise isn't good for anyone.

A good rule when you have a little one—for your partner, certainly, but also for you—is to sleep when the baby sleeps. It's tempting to try to get as much done as possible when the baby is otherwise occupied, and this is fine for you if it helps you feel less stressed. But put off whatever you can. The responsibilities of daily life will always be there, but your hours of uninterrupted sleep are limited. This is especially true for your partner, who needs to be encouraged to rest as much as possible.

*Pooping*

Your newborn came preloaded with poop called meconium. Meconium is made up of amniotic fluid, discarded skin cells and other bits of waste your baby ingested in the womb. You can expect to see meconium, which is thick and tarry, in your baby's diapers for the first few days before the transition to normal poop.

One of the advantages of breastfeeding is that the baby's poop, until solid foods are introduced, is pale in color and has a mild, inoffensive odor. Be prepared, though—there is likely to be lots of it. A baby who gets formula will have poop that is darker in color, thicker and has a stronger smell. Either way, between peeing and pooping you can expect to go through at least 10 diapers a day.

Disposable diapers are easy to deal with, but most are made with plastic that will be landfill for generations to come. Biodegradable diapers are available, although they may be expensive. Cloth diapers are pretty messy to deal with and it can be argued that the laundering they require isn't environmentally kind, either. One nice thing about cloth diapers is you can hire a service to bring you clean ones and take the soiled ones away. Some parents use cloth diapers at home and disposables away from home.

Similarly, you can buy wet wipes for diaper-change cleaning or use washcloths, or use some combination of the two.

## *Crying*

Just about when you and your partner start high-fiving over how well you're handling this whole parenting thing and how lucky you are to have this easy baby, everything changes big time! Your sweet, happy baby has been possessed by a demon spirit that can't be soothed or placated. Crying jags go on for hours, no matter how often you feed, change diapers, burp or walk the halls. You're frustrated, sleep-deprived and sometimes you feel irrationally angry. What's happening?

At around two weeks, normal newborns enter what's been termed the Period of **PURPLE** Crying. The letters stand for:

**The peak of crying**. The crying starts around two weeks, peaks in the second month, then tapers off over months three to five.

**Unexpected**. There's no rhyme or reason to when the crying starts.

**Resists soothing**. Nothing you do makes any difference.

**Pain-like face**. The baby looks to be in pain but isn't.

**Long-lasting**. The baby may cry for five hours a day . . . or more.

**Evening**. Crying is most likely in the late afternoon or evening, even if the baby was perfectly happy all day.

As awful as this period is, it is normal and it does end as the baby's nervous system matures.

This is the time in a baby's life when they are most at risk of being injured by an angry, exhausted parent. You may be horrified to feel rage bubbling up inside you as endless crying pushes you closer to the edge. If you are in danger of losing control, or if you just need a break, this is the time to hand the baby off to your partner or other calmer adult and go for a walk. By taking care of yourself first, you will be in the best form to take care of your child. In fact, there's nothing wrong with gently laying the baby down in a crib, bassinet or another safe place, closing the door and walking away. Not for a long time—you aren't going to neglect your baby or give up on trying to soothe them. But it's better to walk away for a few minutes and catch your breath than to risk harming them.

## *Bathing*

Your newborn doesn't need much cleaning beyond the diaper area. The umbilical stump should be kept as dry as possible to prevent infection, so if more than bottom-wiping is needed it's best to stick with sponge bathing until it falls off. After that, you can do full baths in a baby tub or any container that's big enough for a baby and some water. Lots of parents use the kitchen sink; just be sure to clean it well, both before and after.

    Unless the baby is sweaty or poopy you can just wash with plain water. If you need a little more cleaning power you can use any gentle, mild-smelling soap; it doesn't have to be a special baby product. And you can use one soap on both head and body at this age; shampoo can wait until you've got a full head of hair to work with. Your baby is likely to be very relaxed in a warm bath, which probably brings back happy memories of floating snug and carefree in the womb. Just remember they can't breathe underwater anymore and need to be protected from getting chilled.

## *Umbilical stump*

The umbilical cord was living tissue, and the stump left behind after the cord is cut is living tissue that dies. It will shrivel up and turn black, and a small amount of fluid may leak from the point where it joins your baby's still-living skin.

You'll be given instructions on how to care for it. Basically, you'll wipe away any poop that gets on it and try to keep diapers from rubbing against it (disposable diapers for newborns often leave a space in front for this reason).

Parents used to be told to apply rubbing alcohol to the stump, but this isn't really necessary. Infection is rare but you'll want to check in with your baby's healthcare provider if you notice redness, swelling or smelly discharge.

## *Vaginal discharge*

Sometimes a newborn baby girl will have a little vaginal discharge, either light in color or even a little bloody. Her vulva may also appear red and swollen. This is caused by exposure to mom's hormones before she was born and will gradually clear up.

## *Foreskin care*

If your baby boy has an intact foreskin, it probably won't be very moveable at first. Just wash around it ("clean what's seen") and never use force to retract it. If he's already been circumcised, you'll have been given care instructions.

# Chapter 20:
# Parental care at home

On the one hand, pregnancy and childbirth are normal, natural parts of life and women do it every day. On the other hand, creating a new life and bringing it forth into the world is like having the greatest superpowers ever, and doing it makes your partner a superhero.

Just as some women seem to breeze through pregnancy while others endure nine of the most miserable months of their life, some will be up and fully active right after giving birth while others will undergo an extended period of slow recovery. Your partner will probably fall somewhere in the middle. She's been through a lot, and she deserves some consideration, even more so if there were complications along the way.

With all this attention on your partner's needs, you may feel at times like your own needs are being overlooked, and that's likely to be true for a while. But as your partner recovers from the physical stress of childbirth and you both get better at handling the demands of parenthood, this will get better. You will have a social life again, you'll be able to focus on your career and you'll even get to enjoy time to yourself. Maybe not as much as before—but the trade-off will be well worth it.

## *Her emotions*

It's impossible to predict what your partner's emotional state will be just after the baby is born. Certainly, the amount of support she has, and the amount of sleep she's getting, will have a big influence, as will the continuing ebb and flow of hormones. Overall, a mix of positive and negative emotions is to be expected, as with any major life change. It's very common, though, for new mothers to have a range of bad feelings they may find hard to talk about. Some celebrities are helping overcome the stigma of postpartum mood disorders by openly sharing their own experiences.

*Postpartum blues*

It's estimated that up to 90 percent of all women experience some degree of "baby blues." The blues generally kick in a couple of days after birth, peak within the next few days and then gradually resolve over about two weeks. Your partner may have times when she feels sad, frustrated or angry. She may cry easily and have doubts about her mothering abilities. These feelings come and go, resolve with sleep, exercise or emotional support, and alternate with times when she feels happy and optimistic.

*Postpartum stress syndrome*

The next step up in severity is postpartum stress, which may afflict up to 75 percent of all new mothers. If your partner has postpartum stress she may appear to be coping well, while inside she is eaten up with anxiety and sadness. She may feel disappointed in herself, her baby and the experience of motherhood, and she may worry she isn't up to the job. She may find it very hard to admit she's having these feelings, as that would feel like proof she's not good enough. Hopefully you know your partner well enough to recognize the signs of stress and can offer extra support to help her get through it. Encourage her to talk about her feelings, either to you or to a trusted friend or family member.

## *Postpartum depression*

Postpartum depression affects up to one in every four new mothers. Postpartum depression can be sneaky, either coming on early like postpartum blues or not rearing its ugly head until 18 months later. This form of depression runs much deeper than the blues and can completely destroy your partner's self-esteem and ability to take any pleasure in her baby or her life. If your partner suffers postpartum depression, she may have thoughts of harming herself or the baby—she needs professional care, urgently. She should start with her own healthcare provider to rule out medical conditions that could be contributing to her depression.

*Postpartum anxiety*

Closely related to postpartum depression and sometimes going along with it is postpartum anxiety, which affects up to one in 10 women. This is not the normal anxiety that comes with being a first-time parent. Sometimes the anxiety is generalized, and sometimes it manifests as postpartum panic disorder or postpartum obsessive-compulsive disorder. Women who have experienced anxiety before having a baby are most at risk. Professional help may be needed.

## *Postpartum psychosis*

Fortunately, postpartum psychosis is rare; this severe mental illness is estimated to affect only one or two out of every 1,000 new mothers. Women who were diagnosed as bipolar before pregnancy are at the greatest risk, but any woman can be affected. Psychosis is a break with reality. In the unlikely event, your partner experiences postpartum psychosis she may have frightening mania, crippling depression or both. She may also suffer terrifying delusions and hallucinations, putting her, the new baby and any other children she has in grave danger. Postpartum psychosis is an emergency and requires immediate medical care.

## *Your emotions: Paternal postnatal depression*

Yes, it can happen to you, too. You might not be experiencing the same hormone flow and body changes as your partner, but you are also worrying, stressing and losing sleep. You may be dismayed to find the happiness wearing off and the reality of becoming a father weighing heavily on you. This is incredibly normal; estimates are that up to one in every four new fathers experience some degree of postpartum mood disorder.

If it happens to you, make sure you're getting some time *you* time. Go out for a run or bike ride, or meet up with the guys for a little basketball or a celebratory beer. If you find nothing makes you feel better, don't be afraid to get professional help.

## *Her vagina*

It's been through a lot. If you watched your baby being born you may have doubted your partner's vagina could ever be its old self again, but it's amazingly resilient and will bounce back in time.

After a vaginal delivery she will have bleeding for up to six weeks and her cervix will need time to close completely. Intercourse during this time is not recommended due to the risk of uterine infection. If she had perineal tearing or an episiotomy she will feel pretty sore. Typical comfort measures include ice packs followed by sitz baths, which basically means soaking in a warm bath. She may be advised to encourage healing by laying on the bed with her legs apart and aiming a lamp at the area.

## *Her belly*

Some women are surprised to find they still look pregnant after the baby has been born. This may be partly due to the weight put on during pregnancy, and partly to the stretching and softening of the abdominal muscles. Your partner may notice very distinct separation of the rectus abdominis, the "six-pack" muscles. This is called diastasis recti and usually resolves with time, although in some women the abdominis never fully fuse again.

If your partner had a C-section she will probably have a horizontal incision low on her abdomen. This is known as a "bikini cut" because it's low enough to stay hidden under bikini bottoms. The old school vertical cut up the center of her abdomen is rarely done anymore. Her incision may have been sutured or stapled; staples make for a quick and convenient repair but sutures are less likely to lead to infection or other complications.

If your partner has stretch marks they may be red or purple now. They will fade in color over time and may nearly disappear.

## *Her breasts*

Although they likely grew larger and heavier during pregnancy, your partner's breasts won't actually start producing milk right after the baby is born. She will produce a creamy, nutrient-rich pre-milk called colostrum, though, and the colostrum along with the baby's body fat and fluids accumulated in the womb will carry it through until her milk comes in.

Within a few days her breasts may fill with milk suddenly, becoming large, hard and very tender; this is called engorgement. The best treatment for engorgement is a hungry baby! At first her breasts may fill with far more milk than the baby can drink, and she may be tempted to relieve the pressure by pumping or expressing (pressing with the hands) the excess milk. This can be done just a little if she's really miserable or if her breasts are so hard the baby is having trouble latching on, but it's best to resist the temptation as it gives her breasts the message that more milk is needed. Within a few days, her milk supply will adapt to the baby's appetite and everyone will be happier. If your partner isn't going to be breastfeeding, her milk will still come in and she'll be given instructions on how to proceed.

# **Conclusion**

Having a baby is truly the most natural thing in the world. Whether you thought you were ready or not, now you're on your way. And you will find your way, just like all the generations of men who came before you. Like them, you'll make mistakes. And like them, you'll have moments of parenting brilliance. And in the end, you'll find the rewards of fatherhood far outweigh the hard work and sacrifices involved.

It may seem like there's a lot to know and think about—and there is! But just like your dad, and his dad before that, you'll figure it out. You've got time before the baby comes to get ready, and years afterward to get the hand of this parenting thing. Be strong, be flexible and get ready for the adventure of a lifetime. And remember: you just have to be present.

**Do let us know how this book helped you by leaving a review. This will encourage eager parents to make the right purchase, also I get motivation whenever I hear someone who gets value from what I created.**

**Happy Parenting!**

# Newborn Care Basics:

*Baby Care Tips For New Moms*

*Author*
*Lisa Marshall*

# Introduction

Congratulations on downloading *Newborn Care Tips: Baby Care Tips For New Moms* and thank you for doing so. With as much advice as there is about babies out in the world, this book will be your first step to gain more knowledge about the basics. It is there to help alleviate some of the concerns that you may have as a new parent in those first overwhelming moments. This book will serve as your trusted guide as you watch your baby grow.

The following chapters will discuss the basics regarding newborn care for all parents. Chapter by chapter, it will lead you through the baby's first couple of weeks concerning anything from feeding baby to clothing baby. These chapters include information on bonding, belly button care, and even circumcision without being biased towards anyone's way of raising a baby.

It is the hope that they will be not only informative but that they will be a guide to assuage any fears that may be lingering after the birth of the most precious gift, your baby. It is in those moments, when parents are feeling their most vulnerable, that a handy guide such as this will be most valuable.

It will also show you that there is no one right way. Babies tend to do things at their own pace and are their own human beings with specific preferences. Some babies sleep, and some do not. Some babies like warm milk, and some like it cold. This does not mean that you as a parent are doing anything incorrectly.

There is also some special information for those parents that have decided to take the journey of parenthood through adoption. It is the journey of raising a baby that makes a person a parent, no matter how someone became that parent. Adoption is a wonderful gift to give to a child in need, and one that is most definitely not given lightly.

There are plenty of books on this subject on the market, thanks again for choosing this one! Every effort was made to ensure it is full of as much useful information as possible, please enjoy it!

# Chapter 1:
## Bonding with Baby

As you begin the miraculous journey of caring for your newborn baby, different questions start to arise. This particular chapter hopes to alleviate any questions that you may have concerning bonding with your baby, a very natural and important process that helps the baby grow to become a fully functioning and loving adult. A bond is what makes a family.

Bonding is the attachment that is formed between a newborn baby and its parents. This bond is the one that allows the family to be in tune with one another, responding to needs as necessary. Through this bond, the parent will know when the child needs something, for instance, helping a mom wake up in the middle of the night to feed the child.

A bond works almost like a communication tool between the parents and the baby. Since a newborn is still too young to speak and make their wishes known, forming a bond with its caregiver is the one way in which the baby can express its wishes. As mentioned, parents become more in tune with the baby ensuring that its needs are fulfilled in a timely fashion.

The most surprising thing about bonding with a baby is how much it actually requires. This is a bond that is formed through fulfilling the baby's needs rather than just by seeing the baby for the first time. Of course, that does happen as well, but most of the time a bond just requires good, hard work.

**The Importance of Bonding**

This bond is very important to the development of the newest little bundle of joy. When a baby is born, their brains are ready to learn from the moment they sense the world. Their senses will take in all that is around them and expand the most for the first two years of their life.

Studies have been performed that prove that by the time a baby reaches the age of 3, their brain is 90% the size of an adult brain. What this means is that during those first years, their brain is growing the most, including the wiring that it contains. Bonding and consistent human interaction are what assists the brain in building those very important synapses, or connections, within the brain itself.

It has also been proven that newborns should bond with their fathers, and other family members, besides just mom as is usually expected. Various studies have shown that in infants where the father has taken an interest in interacting with them from the start, the baby's development both mentally and physically was significantly enhanced. Kids are also more successful academically if they start developing a bond with dad from the very beginning.

**How to Bond with Baby**

There are many ways in which the bond with the baby can be enforced. A bond between a baby and its parents can be cultivated from the very beginning even if the baby has to go to the NICU for any reason. Though the bond can be developed between the baby and any of the parents, it will form a little differently in each case as for instance, fathers aren't able to breastfeed which is a great bonding experience for mothers.

Each parent can tailor the bonding experience to themselves and their baby, as obviously not every baby is the same. What may work for one family may not work for another, making the list of possible bonding experiences rather lengthy. One important thing to remember during this experience is to allow it to happen as naturally as possible, there is no need in forcing it.

*Bonding with Mothers*

A bond with the mother can start from the very moment that the baby is born. During a vaginal delivery, this is done through the use of skin to skin contact. When the baby is born, barring any issues, the baby can be placed right on top of mom's chest to begin the skin to skin and feeding time. It has been proven that most babies will root for mom instinctively, moving down or up her chest as needed to find their sustenance.

Nowadays, most hospitals encourage this skin to skin time, and it should definitely be an option that is explored. When taking a tour around the hospital labor and delivery, it is best to ask the hospital on their policies regarding this very precious time. Plenty of hospitals will ensure that parents do not get disturbed by anyone during these vital moments, for up to an hour or two after the birth.

Skin to skin is even something that is a possibility for a mom that has delivered via cesarean section. In instances where the mom has a spinal block or an epidural, barring all complications, nurses or the support purse is able to place the baby by the mother's head during the remaining portion of the surgery. This allows the mom and baby to start getting to know each other before she is able to hold the baby on her own. Once that is a possibility, most likely during recovery, the baby will continue the rest of the bonding process through skin to skin and feeding.

Even in an instance where the laboring mother needs to be placed under general anesthesia, bonding is possible. The timeline of the start of bonding will most likely be pushed back somewhat, but it is still something that can be strived for. It is important to remember to speak with the nurses that are providing the care to ensure that all expectations are met. This will ensure that when the mother is united with the baby, enough bonding time is secured.

From there, whether at home or in the hospital, a mother will have plenty of opportunities to bond with the baby. One of the most common ways in which a baby will start to form that bond is through feeding. That bond will develop whether the baby is breast or formula-fed as it is also about the closeness of the act itself. Babies who are breastfeeding, when awake, will stare in the eyes of their mother. If a baby is bottle-fed, the mother should ensure that she is still providing that closeness. This means that whether bottle-fed or not, a mother should limit doing anything else when she is feeding her baby, but look back into their eyes.

If a mother is breastfeeding, she also has the added benefit of taking what is called a "nursing vacation". This does not mean a vacation from nursing, but rather a weekend-long stay in bed with the baby where the baby is free to explore and nurse on demand. Even if a weekend is not a feasible option, it is a good bonding experience for both mom and the baby to lay beside each other without any clothes and feel closeness.

*Bonding with Fathers*

Contrary to popular belief, newborns also need to start bonding with their father from the very beginning. The original school of thought was that at the very beginning, and even throughout most of childhood, a father was not needed. It was always the mother who took care of the children and the household; therefore, fathers never truly began to bond with their children.

Recent studies, however, have shown that if a child begins the bonding process right away, there are surprising benefits. Those benefits are not only for the baby, but they extend to the father as well. The necessary bonding can begin right after the baby's birth whether the mother has had a c-section or a vaginal delivery in the form of skin to skin.

Much as the mother gets the skin to skin time, it can be the couple's decision to provide that time for the father as well. This can take place still in recovery, or it can take place at a much later time, however, it is something that is encouraged for both parents.

Since there will be family members who would also like to meet the bundle of joy, the father can make the conscious effort to bond with the baby after the baby is settled at home. There are many different ways that this bonding can continue such as through assisting with feeds. A baby will bond through feeding through physical and eye contact, something that the father can also provide.

*Bonding Tips*

There are various ways in which bonding with both parents can continue. Though a baby may be small in the beginning and will more often than not sleep most of the day away, it is important to provide as much contact as possible when the baby is awake or feeding. Both parents can share responsibilities equally if that is at all possible.

As soon as the baby begins to be more aware of their surroundings, parents are encouraged to participate in other stimulation such as through making silly faces or taking walks. Even something as simple as a diaper change, performed by either parent, assists in growing that necessary bond. Some small ways in which parents can bond with their baby include:

- Giving the baby a very gentle massage. This can be done either with a bath or without
- Reading books
- Kiss baby as often as you'd like
- Wearing the baby either out of the house or in while doing chores
- Looking into their eyes
- Sing to the baby
- Sleep close to the baby within the safe sleep practices that will be covered later in the book
- Always respond to the baby's cries promptly
- Play with the baby making facial expression or coos
- Play peek-a-boo
- Create a ritual that will work for just you and the baby. This is something that each parent can have separately with the baby.

As new parents, it is important to bring in a support system around the family. This can be in the form of either hospital staff in the beginning, parents, extended family, or friends. Taking care of a newborn becomes a full-time occupation at the beginning, therefore, a helping hand can only assist the parents in having enough time to spend with their baby.

Family and friends that you surround yourself with should be prepared to help you in any way that you would deem necessary such as through providing meals or helping to clean. Sometimes, it can even be in the form of babysitting at your home so that you can sneak a nap or a shower. Some babies are more demanding than others and taking small breaks such as these could also assist with developing a well-rounded bond.

*A walk*

Taking a walk with your baby can become a great bonding experience. Though the common belief is that babies should not leave the house for at least the first month of their life, that is a false claim. In fact, with the proper precautions, it is something that is encouraged as fresh air can be good for the baby, and the recovering mother.

The belief of not leaving the house started with the idea that babies do not have a developed immune system and parents should wait until at least the baby's first shots. However, this is one of the precautions that parents should take; to stay away from large crowds. Though it is impossible to completely make sure that a baby doesn't get sick, by staying away from large crowds it is something that parents can attempt to prevent.

Second, when going for a walk it is best to ensure that the baby is dressed for the appropriate weather. The rule of thumb would be that you should dress the baby the way that you dress yourself. For example, if you would dress yourself in layers, it is best to do that with the baby as well so that they do not get too cold or overheated.

Lastly, make sure that the baby is kept out of direct sunlight. Since babies cannot use sunblock for at least the first six months of their life, it is best to keep them in a shady area. If going for a walk with a stroller, this is usually pretty easy to do.

*Bonding under unexpected circumstances*

Try as we might, things rarely go according to plan. This is all the truer when it comes to the birth of a baby. No matter the best-laid birth plans that a mother carries to the hospital with her, babies follow what Mother Nature wants. In some instances, a baby may be born needing a little extra help, such as if they are born premature, and end up staying in the Neonatal Intensive Care Unit, or the NICU.

Parents dread hearing those four letters together: NICU. It always brings with it a connotation of fear and helplessness, however, that does not have to be the case. Whether the baby is brought back home right away or whether there is a NICU stay, it still requires the love of its parents to thrive and form a bond. This is a process that may be challenging at first, but plenty of hospital staff will be there to assist along the way.

A bond can be facilitated at the NICU by getting involved, much as in the case of a baby that has gone home. Though the involvement may be small, a parent should always ask to participate in any way that they are able to such as through diaper changes, bathing, or feeding. It has been proven that NICU babies thrive best in kangaroo care, which is where the baby is placed on the chest of a caregiver similar in fashion to the way a kangaroo holds their young.

When a baby is born, it automatically recognizes their mother through its various senses such as sense of smell, touch, and voice. Even if a baby is born premature, they are still able to make this recognition due to having spent its entire life up to that point inside of mom's belly.

Since the sense of smell is one of the most powerful senses and invokes memories, it can be used to help the baby not only form a bond, but also to help it grow and leave the NICU. It is suggested that a mom provide the baby with something that has their smell on. For example, some mothers will either provide a shirt they've been in, or they will sleep with a small piece of fabric that can be placed with the baby.

Talking with your baby is also very important at this stage. This type of bonding in the NICU can involve both parents as the baby has most likely heard dad before being born as well. This would be a good time to purchase baby books and begin reading those while spending time with the baby.

## What may affect bonding

As important as bonding is, there are always those factors in life that will pose some sort of obstacle for the parents and the baby. Most of the factors mentioned are things that are beyond the control of the parents, and most likely, anyone else that is in the same situation.

For instance, perhaps the baby has shown up in the world looking much different than what was expected. This could be due to either the parents have formed some sort of perfect picture of their baby in their head, be it hair or eye color, or sometimes it could be because of a deformity. Though thorough screenings while pregnant can detect most abnormalities, there are those that still surprise the parents and medical staff. It is that surprising that could catch parents off guard making it difficult to move forward right away.

Hormones are raging the moment that a mother has given birth to her child, vaginally or through a c-section, there is no difference. Within the first few days after the birth of the baby, a mother can develop what is called the "baby blues". She may feel down, or weepy, for most of the time. Sometimes, it is also a combination of hormones and pure exhaustion having gone through hours of labor or the recovery of a c-section.

Postpartum depression, which women are now starting to discuss at length and openly, plays a very important role in being able to bond with the baby. A woman will never be able to tell ahead of time whether she will develop postpartum depression, however, if the "baby blues' do not start to go away within a couple of days from giving birth, it is important to reach out for help, even if it is to talk to a regular or the ob-gyn so that they may point you in the direction.

Most doctors now implement a questionnaire that is requested as they see both the mother and the baby, which means that you may end up encountering the same questionnaire multiple times at different doctors. It is important to be as forthcoming as possible so that if an intervention is needed, the help is provided as soon as is possible.

**Common misconceptions**

Even though it is proven that a baby needs to bond with its caregiver, the best of whom being mom and dad, there are always misleading schools of thought when it comes to how parents go about it. With new studies and advancements in medicine and science in general, various bonding methods have been proven to work. Unfortunately, there are still different misconceptions about the process which should be put to rest right here.

*Bonding is instant*

One of the most important pieces of information to remember when it comes to bonding with the baby is that it is not always instantaneous. The common belief is that parents love their baby immeasurably, from the moment that they are born; that they feel that bond right away. Nothing could be further from the truth. In fact, it is quite normal for any parent not to feel that overwhelming sense of rush they've been told happens from the moment they see their baby.

It is also a misconception that the baby itself will bond instantly. As a matter of fact, the reality is that babies do not necessarily care what is happening in the beginning so long as they are fed and allowed to sleep. It isn't until the baby is roughly two to three months will they develop a strong connection to a caregiver. This common misconception stems from observing other animals. For example, a duckling will imprint on the first thing that it sees and follows it around.

Even if that overwhelming feeling of love or bonding doesn't hit right away, that does not mean that it won't eventually happen. As mentioned, there are many ways in which the bond develops between the parents and baby, but it also takes time. Parents cannot get discouraged if they realize that they did not feel that bond right away. Instead, they should continue caring for their newborn as best as they can and allow the bond to form naturally over time. No matter how long it may take, caring for the newborn will facilitate the process.

*Spoiled baby*

Another common misconception when it comes to bonding is that the baby will end up spoiled. This belief is a result of the bonding instinct between the mother and baby that ensures that its needs are met. In order to effectively bond with the baby, it is recommended as much skin to skin time as is possible along with responding to your baby's cues without making them wait too long. This ensures that the baby understands that their needs will be met and that there are people who care about them. Since forming this bond requires the needs of the baby met to their fullest, an old-school mindset is that the baby will end up spoiled.

Now, no doubt there are kids that are actually spoiled out there, however, that is not as a result of bonding with the baby in the very beginning. A newborn cannot be spoiled because they do not yet understand the world the same way that older children do. They should not have to hear the word "no" or even understand its meaning since their needs are very basic. Denying a baby their basic needs that they are asking for, would not only break the bond that needs to form, but it may also irrevocably hurt the child in the long run.

Some of the most common types of myths out there are:

- Let the baby cry a little: the idea behind this is that a baby will cry to manipulate you, therefore, you should let them wait for a little before rushing to their aid to curb such tendencies. Though on average a newborn will cry roughly for three hours a day for at least the first three months of its life, it is not because she is trying to manipulate you. A baby at that age doesn't know how to manipulate yet, she is simply trying to communicate, and the only way in which she can do that is crying. This is the only way to say that she may be uncomfortable, tired, or hungry. It is best to always check, to the best of your ability, what the baby may need. Now, this is not to say that allowing them to cry for a moment will cause them undue harm, such as if there are other siblings involved that need to be taken care of. This is just to say that when possible, provide to the best of your ability so that the baby always knows that someone is there, helping them bond in the process.

- That the baby is being held too much: in fact, there is no such thing as holding your baby too much. As with preemies who respond well to kangaroo care, so it is also with full-term babies. With the development of various carriers and slings, it allows parents and babies to be close to one another. Contrary to what may be believed, especially with this myth, babies do not need their own alone, floor, or blanket time. By allowing the baby to feel secure with you, whether just through cuddling together, or wearing the baby and doing chores together, it helps the baby feel more secure when you are ready to place them on the floor for fun and learning.

- A routine is needed right away: in actuality, a routine isn't something that is needed until the baby is around three months in age, and even then, the routine should be focused mostly around nap times and bedtime. For the first three months, from the moment that the baby is born, the baby will be the one that dictates that routine or schedule of the day and that is how it should be. The baby will be the one that will determine what it needs and when and it is up to the parents to fulfill those needs, as they are very basic. Allowing the baby to connect and develop empathy is something that starts at the very beginning. Allowing the baby to choose the routine for that first couple of months will not spoil the baby in any way but will show it that it matters in this world and that people care.

*Daycare ruins the bond*

Some parents are in a situation where they need to start looking for daycare for their child right away, mostly due to the need to work. Essentially, living expenses have become so high that in many situations both parents have to work out of the house to provide enough income to live off of. There are many different types of daycare options out there, but most of them will require the baby to be dropped off with other caregivers for a good portion of the day.

The common misconception here is that if a baby is put into a daycare situation they will not spend enough time with their parents to be able to form that special bond. Studies have shown, however, that it is not the length of time that forms the bond, but the quality of the time that is spent together. The attachment that a baby is able to form with adoptive parents only helps to solidify the belief that it isn't about the length of time or genetics. It is always about what one does with that time that matters the most.

What this means for the parents is that when they are home with the baby in the morning, evenings, nights, and weekends, they focus solely on their baby and make the time meaningful. That is the time to put away the phone if feeding the baby and set aside the time to play together and make small routines.

**Bonding in History**

Most of the common misconceptions can actually be attributed to Marshall Klaus and John Kennell and their study of bonding and attachment that they performed in 1976. Though the study they performed used a very small sample of mothers and their newborns, they believed that they found the "critical period" of bonding. Specifically, they studied only 28 women who came from a low-income background. They believed based on their study that the best bonding time was the hour after the birth of the baby, much as is with animals.

Not long after, DeChateau, located out of Sweden, decided to study a small group of 62 middle-income mothers. Here, the findings specified that mothers who were allowed to spend more time with their children within 36 hours after their birth behaved much differently towards their newborns. They held their baby's more often, who in turn cried a lot less.

However, though DeChateau, as well as Klaus and Kennell, did show differences in bonding and mothers' actions as dependent upon how often they were able to spend time with their child, Svejda who studied 30 lower-middle-class mothers did not see any difference worth noting.

Though many tried to replicate the results of Klaus and Kennell, no one was able to do so, and it wasn't until 1984 that the two of them decided to re-evaluate what they found. They determined then, that there is not one process that leads to attachment or bonding.

Bonding was then concluded to have a much deeper meaning than anyone was able to study, the belief shifting to the idea that a bond starts forming when the baby is still in the womb. This is why it is said that biological parents can bond with their children, but adoptive parents need to develop an attachment outside of that bond.

Even though the findings were reviewed again and found inconclusive, the damage, as it were, had already been done. With their first findings out in the open, many people started to believe that bonding had to be instantaneous as opposed to something that could take an entire lifetime to make.

## Bonding Cultural Beliefs

Cultural beliefs on bonding have a significant impact on how bonding takes place. Though in most cultures, the birth of a baby is seen as a joyful time, some cultures do not specifically facilitate the bond that needs to develop.

It was always the hunter and gatherer cultures that helped the bond to go due to the very nature of the society as a whole. In these cultures, the baby will spend most of its time with the mother as she works different chores. Most of the time, the baby will be on their mothers back and breastfeeding is encouraged right from the beginning.

In the western world, especially now, these types of cultural norms do not necessarily exist everywhere, and parents must work very hard for the bond that they seek. The western world prides itself on working and in some instances, families need both parents to work. This does not help mothers to bond with their children right from the get-go, with poor maternity plans in place or breastfeeding support which is no longer seen as the norm.

Indeed, the western world needs to work towards the goal of assisting parents in those crucial beginnings, especially when it comes to shifting their thoughts on breastfeeding children. With little to no support, especially outside of the home, mothers tend to give up this practice quite easily even if it was helping them bond with the baby they've known in the womb for nine months.

This cultural shift is beginning to take place, but it is very slow, which means that parents need to stand up to those norms that need to change. Mothers need to stand up for themselves and their right to breastfeed and have support in doing so.

## Bonding with adoptive parents

By its very definition, bonding is something that can only happen between the birth parents and their child, but that does not mean anything bad for adoptive parents.

Adoptive parents get to go through a process that is called attachment. This is a two-way process, unlike bonding which is a one-way process, between the parents and the baby. Attachment tells the child that they matter to the parents, that they will always be there to protect it no matter what. In order for the family to grow with one another, this attachment must be achieved.

Parents can take some steps to ensure that the beginnings with the baby help this attachment to grow as it should:

- Feeding the baby: specifically, feeding the baby when she determined that she's hungry. Let the baby pick the schedule as it allows them to understand that their needs matter and you are willing to put them above your own.
- Eye contact: look into your baby's eyes often. Make contact while you are feeding the baby or playing together, as it facilitates the feeling of closeness. Let the baby look for you and come to you.
- Holding: and this could include anything from holding the baby, kissing, touching, cuddling, giving a small massage. The idea here is to show the baby as much affection as possible. Respond to the baby's cries as quickly as you can.
- Sound: which just means to talk to the baby, sing, read some books. Use a soft tone of voice and if you notice that other sounds startle

your baby, try to minimize them until the baby gets accustomed.

- Playing together: though newborns sleep most of the day, play with them as much as possible such as through peek-a-boo.

Attachment is as important to develop for adoptive parents as bonding is for natural parents. An attachment bond takes a little bit more work on both the parents and the baby, but it can be just as meaning as a bond is. Much like any other parent, adoptive parents will also go through their own emotional struggles and must keep this attachment in perspective.

As much as any parent would like everything to go as smoothly as possible, that is rarely the case. Parents must not get discouraged as the beginnings with a newborn are usually a trying time. Babies, whether adopted or not, will naturally cry for various reasons, but it is how parents react to those cries that will determine the type of bond or attachment that will develop.

One very important thing to remember is that as an adoptive parent, you are not alone. Many parents who adopt their children go through the same processes and worry about mostly the same things. If you find yourself worrying about any part of the process, it is best to reach out to support groups or other parents because at the very least it'll be easier to see that this journey is not a solitary one.

**Takeaway**

Bonding is a process that, though it is natural, is not always something that is instant. Parents that adopt a child have just as much of a chance of bonding with the baby as parents who have had their own baby. Sometimes, bonding is difficult for different reasons, but parents should not give up right away. It is the hard work that is given to the child that builds that bond all parents hope for.

Attachment, much like bonding, is a process that is not always instant, but it is something that is very important for the family to grow together. It is up to the parents to help facilitate a good environment for the attachment to grow, understanding that it will involve hard work, which will be greatly rewarded.

Not all cultures are alike and in some culture the bond is not something that society as a whole bother themselves with. These are the cultural norms that need to be taken down by parents to ensure that each and every generation has the ability to grow into the best people that they can be.

Take the time to make those small bonding or attachment moments mentioned above and take the time for you. Any parent that has asked for help and has rested themselves, is better able to continue caring for their baby in a way that will help the bond or attachment to thrive.

# Chapter 2:
## Feeding a Newborn

Feeding a newborn baby can be quite daunting for some first-time parents. Those feelings are normal to have in the beginning and they can be overcome with practice and patience. When it comes to feeding a baby, there is no one correct way to do it, however, there are guidelines. These guidelines provide safe practices that will work to point new parents in the best direction for their family.

From the moment that a baby is born, there are two options for feeding which include breastfeeding or formula feeding. Feeding any type of solids won't start until the fourth month at the very earliest, and even then, the baby has to meet certain milestones before trying any type of solids. Though parents always look forward to this milestone, it is not one that should be hurried.

Most of the time, the baby will let parents know when they are ready to move on to the next stages of feeding.

Below is an outline of breastfeeding and formula feeding so that parents can make the decision that will work best for them. As with many things, the decision is completely up to the parents and there is no right or wrong answer. Every avenue has its benefits and its downfalls, and all must be evaluated for the best answer. As this topic can be a rather controversial one, it is best to not allow anyone to sway your decision, but rather do what is best for you and your family.

**Breastfeeding**

The American Academy of Pediatrics as well as the American College of Obstetricians and Gynecologists strongly suggest that a baby be strictly breastfed for the first six months of its life.

Their suggestion means that a baby would strictly receive breastmilk, whether straight from the breast or through a bottle, without receiving anything else such as formula, water, or juice.

Though the AAP make breastmilk the recommended source of nourishment for babies, undertaking breastfeeding is a very personal decision. Breastfeeding comes with as many challenges as it does rewards and should be carefully considered. Most people have strong opinions about breastfeeding whether they support it or not, making that something that has to be contended with.

No matter the opinion of the public, breastmilk is a wonderful source of nutrients for the baby. Breastmilk has the perfect balance of all vitamins, proteins, and fats that the baby will require for those first six crucial months of its life. Though breastmilk is forever being studied, it was determined that it is able to adjust itself to what the baby needs at any given time. For example, breastmilk can provide the baby with specific antibodies if the baby starts feeling under the weather. The information for what the baby needs is passed down to the mother through the baby's saliva as it feeds directly from the breast.

In that fashion, breastmilk regulates its supply based on how much and how often the baby eats. Most advocate for breastfeeding on demand which means allowing the baby to sit on the breast however long it wants whenever the baby demands it. Some mothers breastfeed on a schedule, where the baby has put to the breast every three to four hours and nurses for a set amount of time, usually at fifteen minutes on each side.

The method in which the baby is fed will depend, most of the time, on the baby itself. Some babies will adapt a schedule all on their own, and some will demand food more often. One point to remember is that the baby must be fed at night as well until the pediatrician has deemed that the baby gained enough weight. Until the baby at least doubles in weight from their birth weight, they must be woken in the middle of the night, or dream fed at least every three to four hours. This will ensure that the baby stays fed and hydrated allowing them to gain the right amount of weight.

*Breastfeeding obstacles*

The journey of breastfeeding starts right after the baby's birth with the assistance of a nurse, lactation consultant, or a midwife. No matter how the baby enters the world, whether at the hospital, c-section or at home with a midwife, that journey can begin. In most instances, the baby will be put to the breast as soon as the mother is able to hold her baby and take instruction.

It is important to ask as many questions as you can and accept the help that is given while embarking on this journey. As with many things, there may be some obstacles, but they can be overcome if the mother would like to continue with that journey. Some of the most common obstacles and what can be done about them are:

- Pain! Breastfeeding can be a painful process in the beginning as the nipples begin getting used to the baby eating every couple of hours if not sooner. Some homemade remedies can be tried such as soothing the nipples with nipple cream, checking the baby's latch, and air-drying your nipples. Placing some breastmilk on them could also assist them in healing quicker. In a case where the pain does not start to subside, the mother should reach out for additional assistance such as by contacting a lactation consultant.
- The mother doesn't produce enough breastmilk. At first, the breasts provide a liquid

called colostrum which is the most beneficial to the baby by providing it with fat-rich nutrients and immune-boosting antibodies. Since a newborn baby's stomach capacity is no more than the size of a cherry, the baby does not need to consume large amounts of it. Within a couple of days, breastmilk comes in and begins to regulate itself based on the baby's demands. When demand changes so does the mother's supply, however, a fussy baby does not automatically mean that there is not enough supply. As the baby grows it goes through various growth spurts which cause the baby to eat more and more often. It is quite alright to allow the baby to do so without further interfering so long as the baby is still producing enough urine and stools. Studies show that those are the times when women usually stop breastfeeding as they are unaware of the process, whereas they should continue through those harder times. The time to consult a medical professional starts the moment that the baby is no longer gaining weight or producing enough diapers as you do not want the baby to get dehydrated.

- Your baby has the wrong latch. The baby can have an incorrect latch for various reasons such as the mother having inverted or flat nipples, the baby was premature, or the baby has a tongue or lip tie. If the issue is inverted or flat nipples and the baby is unable to grab a good hold of them, there are nipples shields that can be purchased at most drug stores that assist the baby by bringing the nipple to the front. In other cases, a medical professional can be asked to provide assistance by showing either different breastfeeding positions or determining if the baby may need to have a tongue or lip tie resolved. Most babies are able to continue breastfeeding after a lip and tongue procedure without any problems.

- A mother's breasts are leaky or hard. In those cases, not only does breastfeeding become a chore, but it can be painful even if the baby has the proper latch. Great care must be taken to allow the baby to continue latching, but also to prevent inflammation of the breasts cause mastitis which is very painful and can cause infection. In the case of hard and full breasts the baby must be fed more often, or the milk expressed so that it does not build up to cause the inflammation. If a baby is having a hard time latching in that situation, a little milk can be expressed by the mother first to make the latching easier for the baby.

- The mother may miss her body belonging to just her. Breastfeeding a child means that some guidelines still have to be adhered to, much as they did during pregnancy. Though they are not as strict, in some instances it is true that what mom eats so does the baby. That is why it is advised that mothers try and refrain from drinking too much alcohol or caffeine and still stay away from certain foods. After nine months of pregnancy, it is difficult for a mother to imagine having to go through certain restraints again for at least another six months to a year, and those thoughts are quite normal to have.

*Benefits of Breastfeeding*

Breastfeeding comes with as many benefits as it does obstacles. Even if a baby is not breastfed for a full year, since a baby still requires either breastmilk or formula after six months of life, both mother and baby can still reap the rewards of providing breastmilk.

- Breastfeeding has been known to lower the risk of SIDS (Sudden Infant Death Syndrome). Scientists have not been able to secure an answer as to why that is, but studies have shown that fewer babies suffer from SIDS when they are breastfed.

- As mentioned earlier, it allows the bond between mother and baby to form and to stay secure.
- Breastmilk protects the baby against many different diseases such as Type 1 Diabetes and spinal meningitis.
- It has been linked to smarter babies which have been tested through IQ scores later on in life.
- Breastfeeding mitigates the possibility of obesity as the baby gains weight at just the right amount.
- For mothers, there is a benefit of burning extra calories as well as assisting in the contracting of the uterus back to its pre-pregnancy size.

Though there are wonderful benefits to breastfeeding a baby, in some instances that is not an option. Anyone of the obstacles mentioned can hinder a mother's ability to provide breastfeed exclusively, but there is still the option of pumping breastmilk if there is breastmilk available. Of course, this option would not work if the mother was having a hard time actually getting a supply of breastmilk no matter the steps that she chose to do so.

Many mothers choose the route of pumping breastmilk whether they return to work or not, either because they have had trouble breastfeeding (such as the wrong latch), or for personal reasons such as wanting others to be able to care for the baby as well and having the freedom to step away. Pumping is a good way to build up a stash of frozen breastmilk that can be used later down the road.

*Pumping*

Mothers also choose to breast pump if they have to go back to work before the baby is eating regular food. In the United States, the law requires that employers provide a new mother with an appropriate place and ample time to pump milk during the day. It is recommended that a mother pumps every few hours, most choose between three and four hours, to ensure that supply does not dwindle.

When proceeding with pumping, whether exclusively or just at work, the mother can purchase a pump through her health insurance plan if she has one. It should be mentioned that the flanges which attach to the breast are not a one size fit all. Nipples come in all different sizes; therefore, the flanges should be measured to ensure a correct fit. If the flange is the wrong size, it may not suction correctly and either cause pain to the nipple or not stimulate the nipple enough to produce enough of a supply of milk.
Since pumped breastmilk is going to be stored outside of the body, there are some steps that need to be taken to ensure that it is still being provided as fresh as possible.

- Freshly Expressed breastmilk: this is milk that has just been expressed by hand or pump straight into a bottle. It can last on the countertop, at regular room temperature for up to four hours. If it is refrigerated, it can last up to 4 days, so long as the refrigerator is properly cooling. In a freezer, it can last up to 6 months. Though it can be used up to 12 months if it is in a deep freezer, it is best to use it as quickly as possible.
- Thawed milk that was previously frozen: once it is defrosted, it can last up to two hours on a countertop at normal room temperature. Once defrosted, but not brought completely to warmth, it can stand in the refrigerator for up to one day. To ensure that bacteria are not introduced, it can never be refrozen.
- Milk leftover in a bottle from a feeding: it needs to be used within two hours after the baby last ate the bottle. This means that milk that has been defrosted or freshly expressed, cannot be refrigerated or frozen once the baby has started

eating from that bottle even if they do not finish it.

Breastmilk is hard to come by, a woman who has decided to pump can only attest to the hard work that goes into being able to express it and freeze it for later. For this simple fact, it is best to start with a smaller amount until the baby shows the desire to continue eating, as opposed to making a very large bottle where most of it will end up going to waste.

**Formula**

Infant formula has a long history that dates back to the 19$^{th}$ century. In 1865, a chemist named Justus von Liebig is the first to develop and patent commercially available infant formula. It did not become popular until 1958 when it became more accessible to the common mother causing breastfeeding to go out of favor. Since then, the question of whether to breastfeed or use infant formula has been a controversial debate among mothers.

Ultimately, the choice on whether to use infant formula rests solely with the parents of the child and is the best substitute to breastmilk. There are many reasons why parents would decide to use formula instead of breastfeeding, but the reason for its use should not matter to anyone else. Much as with breastfeeding, there are pros and cons with the use of infant formula and barring a situation where infant formula is the only answer, those pros and cons should be considered.

*Formula obstacles*

As breastfeeding comes with its own set of obstacles, so does infant formula.

- Formula and all the accessories needed can be expensive. Since the baby will be eating multiple times throughout the day, that will require many bottles to be purchased ahead of time. On average, the cost of formula is around $0.19 for an ounce which means that for a year of formula the cost will be around $1,700. Parents must also add the aforementioned costs such as bottles and nipples.
- Infant formula must be prepared each time to ensure that it is measured correctly and to the appropriate temperature. This will cause some distress as the baby will likely expect the food to be provided right away. The formula cannot be prepared too hot or, in some instances, too cold due to the baby's preference.
- The formula is harder to digest than breastmilk which means that it is possible for the baby to become constipated and gassy. In the beginning, it is also possible that some cans of formula will end up going to waste due to such issues as parents have to try multiple different

formulas in order to find one that fits their baby best.

- Lastly, the formula doesn't have the same protective properties that breastmilk does. Since breastmilk is tailored to each baby specifically, and colostrum is so full of antibodies, it is not something that infant formula would ever be able to provide.

*Benefits of Infant Formula*

Using infant formula does also come with its benefits even if they are different from the benefits that breastfeeding provides.

- Mother is able to get a break when needed, or even something as simple as being able to run to the store alone, since a family member or caretaker is able to feed the baby as well.
- With infant formula, it is easier to see how much the baby is eating. This can alleviate a lot of

stress that breastfeeding mothers get because they are not sure if the baby is getting enough or gaining enough weight.

- Since all infant formula is regulated to provide the baby with the same benefits, what mother eats doesn't bother the baby. With breastmilk, the mother's diet will affect what the baby eats, therefore, she would need to abstain from things such as alcohol or excessive amounts of caffeine. A mother using infant formula does not have that to worry about.
- Babies that are fed using formula do not need to eat as often as babies that are breastfed. This means, that they do not have to be fed in the middle of the night quite as often or for as long as breastfed babies do. This provides the mother and the baby with more restful sleep.

As with breastmilk, there are certain guidelines when it comes to the making and storage of formula bottles. They must be adhered to as much as possible to mitigate the possibility of any bacteria being introduced.

- Once a container of powder formula has been opened it must be stored in the sealed container (best to use the same one that it comes in) in a dry place to prevent molding.
- The unmixed formula, such as the powder formula, should not be stored in the refrigerator, but rather at room temperature.
- It is best that the powder formula is used within one month of being opened.
- It is possible to make bottles of formula ahead of time as long as they are kept within the refrigerator. Some parents decide to make enough formula to last twenty-four hours, the longest length of time suggested in the guidelines before it needs to be thrown away, by storing formula in a large container in the refrigerator. You can also make one bottle ahead of time so that all you have to worry about is warming up the bottle itself.

- Any prepared or ready-to-feed formula needs to be thrown out within one hour if it has been sitting untouched.
- Any formula, whether prepared or ready-to-feed, needs to be discarded if the baby is not showing any interest in the remaining portion. This will prevent any bacteria from being introduced to the baby.

The formula has had its ups and downs since its invention. With each decade the trend on what was best, whether formula or the breast, changed. At one time, formula was seen as the "rich" way to do it, due to the sheer cost of it all. It still remains a rather costly thing, but it is no longer seen as something that those that are considered rich have to do to show their status.

**Burping**

With feeding comes the wonderful task of burping the baby, a task which many parents fail to do properly. When a baby has not been burped properly, or for the best amount of time, unintended consequences tend to happen.

Most of the time, parents will lay the baby back down much sooner than they should have. This causes the baby to start to spit up or gas. This causes the baby to lose the precious milk or formula that they've been given, starting the process over again. In some instances, the baby will actually wake up screaming because they are in pain from the trapped gas.

Burping is an essential part of the feeding process, no matter how long it might take. Some babies are great at being burped, whereas some babies will require a little more work. Therefore, different burping techniques have been developed to aid parents in deciding which one works best for their baby.

- Over-the-shoulder: this is one of the most common burping techniques. As the name suggests, you put the baby high on your chest with the baby's chin resting on your shoulder. From there, you pat or rub the baby's back gently until they burp.
- Face-down: in this technique, you place the baby face down across your lap, and as above, you gently put or rub their back. You have to make sure that the baby's head is supported on your lap and facing one side so as not to cause any undue harm or possible spit up before the baby has a chance to actually burp.
- Baby exercises: this technique involves a series of different exercises that can be done with the baby that encourage burping. These include leg bicycles or moving legs up and down and in a circular motion.

- Upright: here the baby is sat upright on your lap facing one side. With one hand you would support the baby's head and with the other gently pat or rub their back until they burp.

These are by no means a one-size fit type deal and as parents, you would need to figure out what works best for your baby. Remember, each baby is different and will respond differently to every technique.

Though it may add a couple of more minutes to a feeding session, which at night might feel like forever, it is time well spent. It will ensure that the baby can remain happy for a longer period of time, and in the night or nap time, make sure that they are not woken up too early because of gas pains that could have been avoided.

**Necessary Accessories**

Whether as a family you choose to breastfeed or formula feed the baby, there are certain things that will need to be obtained in order to make feeding not just successful, but also something that can be enjoyed.

*Breast Pump*

Even if the choice has been made to exclusively breastfeed the baby, which means not supplementing with any formula, a breast pump should be either purchased or obtained through the insurance provider. It is now the law in the U.S. that any health insurance that is covering the woman during her pregnancy, has to provide her with a breast pump. Every insurance has its own rulers on how they cover the machine, for example, some will only send it thirty days before the due date, therefore, it is best to contact them for further information.

There are different types of breast pumps out there, and the choice on which to use will be based on the overall need. If a mother is exclusively breastfeeding and staying at home with the baby, she may not need a large and powerful breast pump just to store a couple of ounces of milk in the freezer, but a woman who is working outside the home may need something more powerful.

- Manual pumps: these pumps are operated by hand and work either with the squeeze of a trigger or through sliding a cylinder back and forth. They are usually small, rather inexpensive, and can be purchased at most stores. They are great for convenience, but they will not work well if the mother needs to express large amounts of milk. Not only would that get time-consuming, but it can also become tiring.

- Battery operated: pumps such as these can become a great alternative to the manual breast pump, but still only work best if there is not a large need for pumping more than once a day. Much as the manual pump, it is convenient, but it can become more costly because of the need to keep replacing its batteries. This is the reason that it is recommended only if pumping is restricted to once a day at most.
- Electric pumps: are more powerful and will yield the best results. Electric pumps are recommended for mothers who want to pump more than once a day, either to make a stash because they overproduce or want some milk stored for a rainy day, mothers that work and find themselves in need of pumping while out of the house, or of course, the mother who pumps exclusively for various reasons. They are more expensive than the previous two options, but they may be covered with insurance as mentioned earlier.

Some mothers also look into purchasing second-hand pumps to cut down on the cost, or to have a spare. A spare can come in handy if the mother goes to work daily, or almost daily, and does not want to carry the pump back and forth between home and work as it can become a burden. Before making such a person, it is best to keep in mind that anything that comes in to contact with breastmilk will need to be replaced.

Due to this, it is best to avoid purchasing a manual or battery-operated pumps second-hand, however, since they are run relatively inexpensive, it should not be too troublesome to purchase them new. On the other hand, most brands of electric pumps have parts that can be replaced rather cheaply and the pump itself that never comes in to contact with breastmilk can be sterilized.

Keep in mind that the accessories that come with a pump, even if it is new, need to be replaced from time to time. The manual that is provided with your particular pump will point you in the right direction on when to replace certain parts and where they can be purchased. Though most of those items are inexpensive, especially as compared to purchasing the formula in the long run, it is always best to shop around for the best price as some items do not necessarily have to be name brand.

If a breast pump is obtained, and all the parts for it, you will also need to purchase milk storage bags. There are many options out there as many baby-oriented companies have made their own variations, but they all work mostly the same. There are also bottles designed for milk storage in the freezer, but they do take up more space, therefore, if you do not have a stand-alone freezer you will be using, it is best to purchase bags that can be easily flattened and kept in the freezer in a storage bin or box.

*Bottles*

No matter the way in which the baby will be primarily fed, it is best to purchase at least some bottles. There will be a need for anywhere between four and ten bottles, depending on how the baby is fed. For a baby that is exclusively breastfeeding and may take a bottle only on occasion, you may not need any more than four bottles. However, for a baby that is fed primarily using formula, it is best to have closer to ten.

A baby will eat at least every three to four hours, therefore, the more bottles that are on hand, the less washing that has to be done. In the beginning, bottles have to be sterilized to ensure that as much bacteria as possible is neutralized. The process of sterilization will go on for some time, most of the time until the baby is at least six months of age and its immune system has started to develop.

Nowadays, there are many different types of bottles on the market. There are bottles made of glass and others of plastic. Some are regular bottles with a nipple and a cover, and some have special inserts in order to become anti-colic. If making the purchase of bottles before the baby is born, it is best to purchase the minimum and if at all possible, at least one of each type. This way, if the baby doesn't take to one type of bottle, a lot of money has not been wasted.

*Bottle warmer*

Though a bottle warmer is not always a necessary item, it is one that becomes quite handy in the long run. A baby's bottle, whether it provides formula or breastmilk, cannot be made too warm. In some instances, a baby will also not take a bottle that is too cold just because of personal preference.

Using the microwave is not something that is highly advised for either breastmilk or formula. First and foremost, microwaving breastmilk will reduce the number of nutrients that are found within and which the baby sorely needs. Secondly, whether it is breastmilk or formula, a microwave causes hot pockets of liquid to form within the bottle instead of uniformly warming it up. This may cause the baby to be burned while they are drinking the milk.

A bottle warmer is the easiest way to warm a bottle to the precise temperature that would be good for the baby. Most of these warmers use steam to warm the bottle whether it is frozen breastmilk or formula in need of warming.

As mentioned, this is not a strictly necessary item, however, it does make things a little easier. Without a bottle warmer it is necessary to find other ways in which to warm a bottle such as thawing frozen breastmilk and warming the bottle on the stove. The same would go for formula since it is usually mixed with cold water. If you feel that the stove may be an easier alternative, the bottle warmer can be skipped altogether. It is also an item that can be purchased later once you realize you may actually prefer that method to the stove.

*Nursing pillow*

Many breastfeeding mothers choose to purchase a breastfeeding pillow. Usually, this type of pillow is in a "C" shape and will sit comfortably around the mother's midsection. A good and supportive nursing pillow will actually assist the baby to get a good latch. It also has been known to help the mother by taking the strain off the arms and back or shoulders by having to hold the baby in the right position. The pillow will actually bring the baby to the perfect height for feeding.

Some mothers who do not breastfeed also choose to use such a pillow as it helps hold the baby in the right position to take a bottle, easing the strain on the hand and back.

A nursing pillow, such as a Boppy, is also used to help the baby do "tummy time". Once the baby is a little older and is curiously looking around, one of these pillows can be placed on a floor with the baby on its stomach to help them lift their heads and explore their surroundings making such a pillow useful in the long run besides just feeding.

*To Go Items*

Unless you plan on becoming a hermit, it is best to take the baby outside even for smaller walks around the park. Until the baby is able to sit at a table and eat what the parents eat, which may be some time, it is best to bring along a few things that may assist in feeding the baby outside the home.

- Nursing cover; If you are breastfeeding your baby and are not comfortable on the outside, it is best to bring a nursing cover. There are also covers out there that have multiple uses, so you are not just bringing along one extra thing. Some will actually work to cover the infant car seat part of a stroller, allowing the baby to go for a ride in peace without prying outside of the outside world.
- Bottle cooler: this can be used both by mothers who breastfeed and formula feed. Some mothers are not comfortable breastfeeding outside the home and choose to bring bottled breastmilk instead. Whichever you choose to use to feed your baby, a cooler for bottles can become handy as a way to store them. Remember, breastmilk does not have to be cooled for at least a couple of hours if it is fresh, but if you are going to be outside longer it may be best to bring an insulated cooler. This could work for formula as

well as some parents choose to take with them prefilled bottles of water. An insulated cooler could actually keep the bottles warmer to the temperature that the baby will be comfortable drinking.

- Formula dispenser: as the name specifies, this is for formula-fed babies, though some parents use these for snacks later as well. These dispensers usually have a couple of compartments where you can prefill specific amounts of formula to fill with water later. Though this can be substituted with small baggies, it makes pouring the formula into the bottle without a scooper that much easier. They are also not that expensive so as to break the bank.

These are just some small suggestions to help make a trip out of the house easier. When leaving home with a baby plenty already has to get packed and having a small list handy is a good idea. That way, you do not find yourself running around to a store trying to find formula because you may not have grabbed any.

## Takeaway

How to feed a newborn is a decision that the parents have to come into agreement on, as breastfeeding requires a lot of support. Parents also have to be prepared that sometimes even the best-laid plans don't go accordingly. When it comes to feeding that happens quite often and there is nothing wrong with changing your mind to something else that would work for the family.

If breastfeeding is just not the ideal choice, the formula has been developed as the most practical and best alternative which offers more or less the same nutrients that breastmilk would. Though there is a bigger push for breastfeeding nowadays for breastfeeding, it by no means signifies that parents are doing anything incorrectly if they choose to either start with or move on to using formula instead.

As with many things in life, there will be those that discuss the merits of one over the other and not necessarily in the privacy of their own home. Parents need not worry about what others think and instead focus on ensuring that their baby is fed, no matter which way that may be. Fed is best, as they now say, and that is just how as it should be. Sooner or later, all babies will start to eat solids, making the whole discussion of breast vs formula a moot point. As long as all babies are allowed to thrive up until that moment is all that matters in the long run.

# Chapter 3:
## Newborn Sleep

The sleep of a newborn is the most elusive thing that there is. It is one of the things that concerns parents the most, mostly because they would like to sleep, exhausted as they are from taking care of a newborn baby. It is fretted about by sleep-deprived caretakers straight from the beginning, especially since newborns do not sleep a lot by their very nature of being newborns. On average, in the first year, parents lose around fifty hours of precious sleep, which is why this topic is such a tense one and parents will do anything for a wink of sleep.

What's most important to remember here, before getting started, is that every newborn is different in their own way. Some sleep better than others and it does not do well for anyone to compare one baby to another. Even among siblings, the changes in sleep patterns can be quite drastic and, unfortunately for the parents, there is no one right answer to what would make a baby sleep better.

Some guidelines can be provided that will assist you, as the parent, in making the best decisions for your family, from safe sleep practices, to where babies can sleep, and if a schedule is at all a feasible option for a newborn, or whether that is something that will have to wait.

## General Sleep Information

Generally speaking, a newborn will sleep most of the day, somewhere between 14 and 17 hours in 24 hours, waking only for a diaper change and feeding. Some babies may even sleep as much as 18 or 19 hours. Since babies have small stomachs and are still getting used to the outside world, they don't sleep for long periods of time.

Breastfed babies tend to wake quicker, somewhere around two to three hours, whereas babies that are formula-fed wake somewhere between three and four hours. It should also be mentioned that in the first few weeks of life, babies should be fed at the same intervals throughout the night even if the baby is showing signs of sleeping longer. This is important to ensure that the baby gains the proper amount of weight within the first few weeks of life. A pediatrician would best be able to advise on when the baby no longer needs to be fed during the night if they continue sleeping longer.

Same as adults, babies have different stages of sleep: REM, or rapid eye movement, and non-REM sleep. REM sleep is the lighter of the two, where dreaming and eye movement occurs. Even though babies sleep for most of the day in the beginning, at least half of their sleep time is actually spent in REM sleep.

Non-REM sleep has four stages for both adults and babies, and they are listed below:

1. This is the initial stage where most of the dozing off happens. Eyes get droopy and tend to open and close.
2. Sleep is still light at this stage and the baby is easy to startle.
3. A deep sleep where the baby is quiet and does not move.
4. In this stage, sleep is very deep, and the baby won't move at all.

It is in those moments that parents question whether they will ever sleep again. The simple answer is that yes, sleep will finally come! Even if the baby takes longer than parents would like, they will eventually sleep for longer intervals. In the meantime, it is best to review some of the tips presented here.

**Safe Sleep**

*Guidelines*

With as much as babies sleep, it is the parents' obligation to ensure that the baby sleeps is in a safe environment to minimize the risk of SIDS. Safe sleep is of the utmost importance as on average, there are around 3,500 sleep-related deaths in the U.S. alone.

When it comes to safe sleep, there are four basic things to remember:

1.      The baby needs to sleep on his back. This is a recommendation until the baby is at least one year of age at which point they should be mobile enough on their own to change positions without getting hurt. The baby should be dressed in pajamas that do not have any loose pieces and will not cover the baby's head. Until the baby is able to roll on their own, they can be swaddled to ensure that they are kept warm, but not overheated. There are plenty of different swaddles on the market, however, the rule of thumb is to ensure that the baby's face will not be covered, and they

will not be able to roll in their sleep in it. If a baby isn't swaddled and starts to roll over on to their side or stomach, it is perfectly all right to move the baby back on to their back while they sleep. In 2015, the CDC performed a study and found that one in every five mothers report that they put their baby to sleep either on its stomach or side, as is not advised.

2.   The baby requires a firm sleep surface. This could consist of a firm mattress that is placed inside a safety-approved crib or a bassinet designed for overnight sleep. A baby should never be placed anywhere that is soft or in a crib with bumpers attached. Soft mattresses and bumpers proved to be a suffocation hazard as a baby can unknowingly press their nose into the bedding without being able to move themselves back into the correct sleeping position.

3.   Any soft bedding such as blankets, pillows, or comforters should be removed. Much as a soft mattress or crib bumpers, any loose items around the crib like blankets and pillows are a suffocation hazard to the baby. In the beginning, the baby will not have the ability to move things away from their face should it get covered. If the baby has something within their reach, they are liable to pull it towards themselves without being able to free their nose or mouth. To put it into perspective, the CDC has found that around 39% of mothers state they use some sort of soft

bedding in their baby's sleep space even though it has been deemed an unsafe practice.

4. Baby should share the parents' bedroom, but not their actual bed. Though companies have designed ways for the baby to join their parents in bed, it is still safest to have the baby in their own space. If parents are not comfortable putting the baby into their own crib until the baby is older, there are regular and bed-side bassinets that can be purchased. They are smaller than a full crib and can be easily reached in the middle of the night. In this fashion, the baby has their own space preventing any possibility of suffocation due to either the parents rolling on to the baby inadvertently or covering the baby with either comforters or pillows.

*Safe Space*

Along with safe sleep comes the choice of where the baby should sleep as parents do have a couple of options. The key is to ensure that the baby will stay safe during the night and be comfortable.

- The crib: is the most common choice by parents, not just in the U.S., but all over the world. There are many different options and looks such as metal or wooden, black or white. The size of a crib is perfect for a nursery or bedroom but will allow the baby to use it for some time. The crib is designed in a way that allows the mattress to be lowered, but because of the bars that make up the crib stops the baby from rolling out. It is, however, not a portable option at all and does take up quite a bit of space if living conditions are tight.

- Bassinet: this is a much smaller version of a crib, which can only be used for a baby that has not rolled over or sat up yet. It is much more portable and can be moved from room to room or to another house if need be but cannot be used for as long as a crib and another option will need to be found once the baby outgrows this. To some parents, this is an unnecessary expense.

- A cradle: this sleep space is even smaller than a bassinet but has the added option of a rocking motion. Since they are smaller than a crib and bassinet, they too are very portable and help with putting the baby to sleep, but the baby will outgrow this option in a blink of an eye.

- Co-Sleeper: a great option for parents who would like to co-sleep but minimize the risk of SIDS or asphyxiation. A co-sleeper is designed to mimic a bassinet where one of the sides gets removed and placed along the side of the bed. This provides easy access to the newborn and is even encouraged for breastfeeding mothers. Of course, like a bassinet, the co-sleeper will become too small for the baby in a very short amount of time.

- The play yard or pack-and-play: is a very popular option especially for parents that are on a budget. They are roughly the size of a crib but can be broken down and made portable. Most of them are on at least two wheels, which makes it easier to bring from one room to another. Since they are almost the same size as a crib, with a mattress that is low to the ground, it can be used for a longer period of time than a bassinet, but still not as long as a crib. There is the chance that by the time the baby outgrows this option, they can be moved into a regular toddler bed.

- Baby swing: though many parents swear by having a sling for their child, this is an item that requires a lot of research. Each brand and type of swing has its own specifications, and some are not recommended for newborns. Most are not recommended for sleep, especially through the night, therefore, though it might be a great item to have in order to be able to place the baby somewhere, it is not something that would be recommended for sleep through the night.

Scientific studies have determined the best ways for a baby to be placed down for sleep whether it is for a nap or bedtime. The rule of thumb is to ensure that the baby is always placed on its back, until it can turn on its own, and does not have anything loose around it such as comforters or blankets. There are many options out there for where to put the baby down to sleep, which will not necessarily all work for each family. Based on the information presented above, it is best to continue doing research to determine what works best for your family.

It is understandable that not all families would like to use a crib, which makes bassinets a better option. For parents who would like their baby close and like the idea of sharing a space, the co-sleeper becomes a great solution. Funds also play a big role in what you would choose for your family. If you have a bit more to work with, or you know someone could assist such as by purchasing a gift at a baby shower, you can use both the bassinet and crib. If you want one stable place a baby can use for a while, maybe a crib that converts into a toddler bed is the best answer.

Whichever you choose to work with, you just have to remember the safe sleep practices and do further research on the item you intend to obtain. Some items such as cribs or pack-and-plays have expiration dates where they are only certified as safe until that day has passed, same as car seats. As mentioned, some swings cannot be used with babies until they reach a certain weight or height requirement, therefore, it is best to ensure you know exactly what you are purchasing and that your baby will be safe.

**Getting Baby on Schedule**

The idea of a schedule is one that is debated amongst parents, however, in the beginning, it is the baby that will end up setting the schedule throughout the day. Most of the time, that schedule will be eating, sleep, then poop over and over again, in roughly two to four-hour intervals. Plenty of times, however, babies confuse their day and night with one another. It is in those times that attempting to set some sort of schedule that could be continued as the baby grows, is of vital importance.

Within the first two weeks of the baby's life, a routine isn't the most important part so much as allowing the baby to understand the difference between day and night. As mentioned, babies tend to confuse the two, therefore, it is up to the parents to help the baby distinguish. This can be done simply by making small routines around different times of the day. Those small routines are the ones that will help the baby make the connection between what is night and what is the day.

A possible day time routine:
- Opening up the blinds
- Turning on as many lights as needed
- Allowing for ample noise

- Small amounts of playtime during awake time
- Rousing the baby fully before feeding
- Do not allow for stretches of sleep that are too long, meaning to still feed the baby within two to three hours so the longer stretches happen at night.
- 
- A possible nighttime routine:
- Quieting the house
- Closing the blinds and turning down any bright lights
- A small bedtime routine to consist of a bath, book reading, and snuggle time
- Avoiding any stimulating activity
- Feed the baby when they wake, but avoid turning on any bright lights

When the baby is roughly a month old, it is best to start implementing a routine that will revolve around times of the day. Most of the same suggestions from above can be kept within this routine, but now implementing an actual bedtime will benefit both the baby and the parents in the long run. There is really no set time in which things should happen as each family and its needs are different, therefore, there is no one right answer. It is best to evaluate possible bedtimes or nap times as they would coincide with the parents already existing obligations such as work or school.

What should be avoided at such a young age is sleep training your baby. A newborn is not yet old enough to understand sleep patterns and has not taught themselves how to self-sooth. Parents must first teach the baby how to self-soothe before they can try and sleep train a baby a couple of months down the road.

The idea is to lay down the foundations in the very beginning for good sleep later on. There is technically nothing getting in the parents' way of teaching their baby how to sleep through the night by around three months of age, though parents do have to also understand that this process may take a little longer than is desired.

**Sleep Problems**

Most parents want to know the signs of sleep problems and what to do about them, however, what parents usually assume is a problem is generally a normal part of infant sleep patterns. Some of the most common patterns that parents assume are issues include:

1. The baby waking more at night, whether they slept through the night or not. Though this may prove problematic, especially for the parents who will start to lack sleep throughout that time, this is quite normal. Usually, this happens around the time a baby is going through a growth spurt and require more food to grow. The baby with a newborn, there is no real solution to this as the baby does need more food. In some instances, it could be solved by providing nourishment that will sustain the baby longer, such as supplementing with formula or talking to the pediatrician about other options.

2.     The baby needing someone to be present when they fall asleep. This could mean that the baby requires to be rocked to sleep or the parent sitting next to them. Again, this is a normal phenomenon. For nine months, or around there, the baby has been inside of mom, kept warm by her body. It is a strange world to be on the outside, it is colder and most of the time noisier as well. Most of the time, this will resolve on its own as the baby grows and gets accustomed to life on the outside. One possible solution parents could try is to work with different swaddles or rockers.

**Sleep Accessories**

*Monitors*

With the development of new technology, came the era of monitors. No longer do parents have to guess whether their baby is sleeping or not, there are various monitors that allow caretakers to see or hear the baby from another room. Plenty more have been developed which provide further information such as whether the baby is breathing.

The choice on which ones to purchase lies solely with the parents and what options fit the family best. There are some important points to remember when choosing a monitor, besides the type, such as:

- Audio monitors – these are relatively inexpensive monitors that provide only audio feedback. In most instances, the audio goes both ways, allowing parents to sooth the baby before they reach it. Most of these are also equipped with a light-up option, which means that as the baby makes noise that the monitor picks up, it will also light up based on the intensity of the noise.
- Audio and Video monitors – monitors such as these are also equipped with a small camera that can be mounted on a wall or set up on a surface. They are either in black and white or color and provide not just the sound of the baby, but a visual as well. They are a tad more expensive than the regular audio monitors but provide

parents with the extra security of seeing their baby sleep soundly. It allows the parents or a caretaker to ensure that the baby hasn't moved, twisted, or otherwise found themselves in a predicament that may be dangerous.

- Wireless network monitors – these are digital monitors that work off an existing wireless connection. The receiver, instead of a small screen, is a device that works off the wireless network such as a computer, tablet, or phone. Since the receiver can be a tablet or a phone, it allows the parents to see their baby from further away, so long as there is an internet connection.
- Movement monitors – are designed specifically to alert parents if their baby has not moved for more than twenty seconds or so and are a little more on the costly side. In order to be effective, this type of monitor comes equipped with a motion sensor pad that is slipped underneath the mattress. It is designed to be sensitive enough to feel the baby's breathing and other movements. Besides monitors that come

with pads underneath the mattress, there are others that are in the form of a sock that the baby wears overnight. There have been no studies performed on whether they are any more effective in the prevention of SIDS and have been formally recommended by neither AAP nor NIH (National Institute of Health).

Though the monitors that are available to parents nowadays are as fancy as they can get, by alerting to troublesome breathing or simply when the baby has woken, there are many people out there that are opting out of the use of baby monitors. Of course, to any new parent, the technology sounds amazing and unbelievably helpful, however, many soon find out that it is not all it is cracked up to be.

Babies will make noise no matter what, especially when they are sleeping, meaning that the monitor will pick up every breath, hiccup, or gurgle that a baby makes, waking parents more often than it should. Movement monitors tend to malfunction, or those with socks slip off as the baby moves in its sleep, again, rousing parents unintentionally, as well as scaring them in the process. It is due to those simple facts that parents are beginning to ditch their monitors. They found themselves rushing in too many times, even if the baby wasn't awake and reacting prematurely.

*Swaddles*

Swaddling a baby means to wrap the baby tightly in a blanket or special swaddle which are currently out on the market. There are a couple of good reasons why swaddling is prominent.
- Stops the baby from being scared by their own startle reflex which can last even up to 6 months.
- Studies have been performed which have found that the act of swaddling a baby could actually help prevent SIDS.

- Keeps the baby warm when the baby cannot use a blanket since anything soft in the crib is not advisable.
- May help to calm the baby. Some parents have found that their baby is much easier to put to sleep when they've been swaddled.

If the baby came into the world at a hospital, you will see the nurses come and swaddle the baby. Before leaving the hospital, it is best to get pointers from those nurses on how to best swaddle a baby and they would be very happy to oblige. It is best to ensure that you are swaddling correctly before you bring your baby home and put them to bed. When using a blanket as a swaddle, ensure that you are following the correct swaddling steps.

- Use a square blanket that has been made for swaddling. Lay the blanket down on a flat surface and fold down the top corner.

- Lay the baby down on their back and ensure that the top part of the blanket is at shoulder height.
- Place the baby's left arm down, then pull the corner of the blanket nearest the left hand over the arms and the chest of the baby, then tuck the edge under their back on the right side.
- Next, bring down the baby's right arm and pull the corner nearest the right hand over the arm and chest and tuck it in on the left side.
- Twist the bottom of the blanket and tuck it behind the baby, leaving enough room for the baby to bend both their legs out naturally. This is done to ensure that the baby does not develop hip dysplasia.

Though swaddling is a practice that has been taking place for millennia, it is still best to be advised on all the aspects of the practice before making the decision to continue the process beyond the hospital stay.

- Opposite to what most parents think, a baby does not have to be swaddled. If you find that your baby has no trouble falling asleep and staying asleep without a swaddle, do not bother continuing on with the process. This will only lead to the issue of having to break the habit later.
- Make certain that you put the baby to sleep on their back. In turn, swaddling should stop the moment that the baby shows any signs of turning over on to their tummy. If a baby were to find itself in that position, they would have trouble lifting their head enough to be able to breathe comfortably.
- Though the baby's legs need to have some freedom of movement to ensure correct development, you have to make sure that the swaddle is nice and snug and cannot come loose. A loose swaddle could pose a suffocation hazard.

Due to these different criteria, different swaddles have been developed to help make the process easier. There are many different swaddles out there, therefore, some research and trial and error may be necessary as not all babies will take to the same swaddle. The best thing to keep in mind is to use a swaddle that will allow the baby to move around their legs and hips.

No matter the type of swaddle used, or even if it's just a blanket, it is best to take into consideration all of the options that are out there. Also, as the caregivers, you have to remember that a swaddle cannot be used forever, even if it makes bedtime much easier. A baby will start to roll sooner or later, and it is at that time they will need to have more freedom while sleeping to ensure that they do not run into the risk of suffocation.

*Other Accessories*

Besides accessories such as monitors or swaddles, other items have been developed that are said to help the baby sleep. There is no written rule that states that these must be purchased, and in some instances, parents may even want to think twice about doing so.

The first item to be mentioned is a soother whether it uses noise or vibrations. Some of these come as combination soothers, which means that the item does both white background noise and vibration. There are also plenty out there that do either one or the other. Most parents will gravitate towards a white noise machine, believing that it will help drown out the noise of the rest of the house, allowing the baby to doze off and stay asleep.

There is even an entire bassinet developed which gently rocks the baby, makes a white noise of some sort and vibrates helping the baby fall asleep. Another bassinet was developed to mimic a ride in the car where it is said babies fall asleep the best.

Though these items may work wonders, they are also something a baby can get very used to and have trouble falling asleep without. This may become problematic as the baby grows and it is clear that they should no longer have to use sleep aids, or they've simply outgrown the item. For example, the bassinet mentioned above will one day be something that a baby outgrows. Since it had been doing most of the work for the parents when it comes to putting the baby to sleep for the night, it will not be an easy process breaking that habit. It may be best to teach the baby how to self soothe from early on, even if it means that there may be some hours of lost sleep.

One more item that is worth mentioning here is a humidifier or an essential oil diffuser; some have even been combined. A humidifier that is used to bring more moisture into the area can be very helpful around dry seasons. They assist the baby to breathe a little easier during those times, making sleep a more comfortable process. If the humidifier has an option to be used as an essential oil diffuser, it becomes an added bonus

**Sleep outside the home**

Neither parents nor the baby can be expected to remain indoors until the child is older. Life continues on, and especially when there are older siblings involved, parents will find that the baby needs to start leaving the house with them right away.

Since, as mentioned earlier, babies sleep most of the time their first few weeks of life, when a baby leaves the house, they will need somewhere to continue on their slumber which is so very important in the beginning.

The length of the trip will determine the best options for a baby, with shorter trips obviously needing less.

- Infant car seat: when leaving the home, to go on a short trip such as a store or to visit a friend or relative, parents will need to take the baby in a car seat. A majority of parents will use an infant cart seat. This type of car seat has a base that has been pre-installed into the car and that can be clipped into the base or into a stroller. This makes it easier to move baby from one place to another, especially if there are a couple of tips in between, such as running errands. A baby can safely slumber in their seat while they are being moved between the car and either store or home. It is, however, important to remember that when going on long car trips, a baby needs to be removed from their seat every so often. Also, an infant car seat should only be used when clipped into either a car or the stroller so that it sits at the optimal angle. Babies are at risk for asphyxiation if they are left in their car seat which is set down for example, on the floor, without the base or the stroller.

- Stroller: some strollers come with either an attached or built-in bassinet. This means that the stroller fully reclines in a laydown position allowing a newborn to sleep laying down much like they would in an actual bassinet or crib. It is convenient if you are staying in one spot for a long period of time, such as if you are going for a walk or a shopping mall. This does not allow for an easy transfer from car to store or home, but it does provide the baby with a safe and flat way of sleeping. Something like this can also be used if you are visiting someone and setting up the stroller instead of a pack-and-play as an example.

- Travel beds: besides the pack-and-play that has been mentioned already, there are smaller portable travel beds out there. Some are even disguised as a diaper bag with just as many pockets to work as both. These are strictly for the newborn as they are relatively small in comparison to even a real bassinet. They do allow the convenience of being able to put the baby down anywhere, whether it's just outside the home, at someone's house, the airport, plane, or hotel. The possibilities with such a bed, so long as space is provided, are endless.

Newborn babies sleep almost anywhere, they just have to be provided with a safe space to do so. For short trips, an infant car seat is perfect especially when running errands and the baby will need to be moved between the car and a store repeatedly within a short length of time. Car seats, however, cannot be used as nap space if they are brought inside and placed anywhere but the stroller or base they are designed for.

There are, of course, other options such as the stroller itself or a travel bed designed specifically to allow the baby to lay in a flat position as is dictated by safe sleep practices.

## Takeaway

Unfortunately, there is no one right answer for the way a baby does or does not sleep, whether they should be monitored while they do, whether they should be swaddled or not, or what actions to take if parents feel there is a problem.

Things to remember are that sleep safe is the most important aspect of putting the baby down to sleep, whether they sleep through the night or not. Most newborns will not be sleeping through the night for a couple of months, and that does not mean there is anything wrong. Their small stomachs mean that they will get hungry faster and it is best to provide them with whatever they need at the moment.

In most instances, it becomes a trial error on the part of the parents. It is, however, not recommended to sleep train a newborn. Sleep training, and there are many schools of thought on this, is something that can take place at a later time when the baby has gotten older and understands more of its world. For now, at the newborn stage, if the baby requires just extra food or more cuddles, parents should focus on providing that the best that they can. One day the baby will be older, a toddler, teenager, or grown-up, and will no longer need that extra care to get to sleep.

# Chapter 4:
## Cleaning Baby

Another tip to parents in the long journey of caring for their newborn is cleaning the baby, which can be either a fun experience or one that parents find daunting. A baby's first bath becomes a major milestone for parents, but it comes with many uncertainties. With so many bathing options out there, as well as advice on best practices, it can quickly become very overwhelming. The hope here is to put some of that to rest.

First and foremost, it is best to keep in mind that a bath should become a pleasant experience, even if in the beginning the baby may appear not to like it all that much. It is a chance for the baby to bond with its parents as this is a task that can be performed by either parent. In some situations, if a mother is breastfeeding, this is something that can be left for the dad to do so that he too can be as involved as possible.

Babies tend to feel safer in the arms of their dad which is what helps the two of them bond. Dad can make bath time as additional time that he gets to spend with the baby, especially if the dad is the one that is working outside of the home mostly.

**Top and Tail**

Topping and tailing refer to washing the baby's head, neck, hands, and bottom. Most of the time it is a process that is employed when the baby's umbilical cord has not fallen off and parents do not want to submerge the baby in water to give it a bath.

Some parents also choose to continue this process in between baths as baby's do not require baths as many times throughout the week as an adult.

Since baby's do not move around as much, and therefore, do not sweat as much, unless necessary for others reason (such as a really bad diaper) on average babies get baths around two to three times in a week. There are some simple steps for this process:

1. Before starting to undress the baby, make sure that you have everything in hand such as a clean diaper, clothes, a towel, a soft cotton rag for washing, and that the room is sufficiently warm.
2. Only a small bowl of water is needed for this process. The water should not be too hot or too cold. If need be, check the water temperature with your elbow as it is a good indicator of how the baby will feel the temperature of the water.
3. After the baby is undressed, it is best to leave the baby on top of a soft towel so that she can be dried right away and kept from getting too cold.
4. Dampening the soft cotton rag, begin with the face using soft and gentle touches, working your way down, and covering the baby as you go.
5. Some parents decide to use gentle baby soap on the genitals and bottom to ensure thorough cleanliness from any poop that the baby may have done.
6. Once you consider the baby to be cleaned, she can be placed back into a diaper and the chosen outfit to keep warm.

The directions above can be used as a general guideline and may be adjusted based on the needs of the situation or the baby. Parents will find that this process will become intuitive with practice.

**First Bath**

Technically, a baby's first bath would be given at the hospital by the nurse, who can also show how the process is done having had many years of practice. Each hospital has different practices when it comes to a first bath, so it is best to ask ahead of time in case you would like to do something different.

In some hospitals, a baby's first bath is given as soon as possible since the baby is coated in different fluids upon entry into the world. However, there are parents that have been choosing to delay that bath at the hospital for up to 48 hours. This decision is made based on the recommendation of doctors who have provided the following information.

- Reduces the risk of infection: this is because delaying the bath leaves the baby covered in what is called vernix in which they are born. Vernix is a white substance that is made up of skin cells which the baby made while they were developing in utero and this coating actually works as an antibiotic ointment, warding off bacteria.
- Assists in stabilizing blood sugar: when the baby is cut off from the placenta, it loses that which had stabilized their blood sugar all of that time. When placed in a bath, babies tend to get stressed which causes the release of hormones which cause blood sugar to drop, a dangerous thing in an infant.
- Helps with temperature control: in some instances, bathing the baby soon causes the baby to go into hypothermia because they are unable to

control their own body temperature when they are born. This is also why babies are kept bundled up or under heat lamps in the hospital.

- Improved bonding and breastfeeding: studies have shown that babies tend to do better with bonding and breastfeeding when they are allowed to stay with their mother without the intervention of medical procedures. In a hospital, a bath would also be called a medical procedure, and it is one that can wait for those precious first hours.
- Moisturizer: vernix works like a natural moisturizer for the skin. Bathing the baby will only remove that moisturizer and it cannot be substituted with anything else.
- Parent special time: by allowing the mother to recover from her ordeal, she is able to participate in that special time between the baby and caregiver. If she would like this to take place at the hospital, the nurse is also there to assist and provide guidance.

The bath that is given to a baby in the hospital as a first bath, will not necessarily appear the same as it does at home. This type of bath is usually what has been described above as a top and tail. Since the baby's umbilical stump still remains attached, the baby cannot be submerged. This also allows the parents to have that special first bath at home if this is not something that they were able to participate in at the hospital.

The first bath at home has become almost a rite of passage, a big milestone for a baby, the moment that parents feel their baby is ready. There are no right answers as to when the baby may be ready, but most parents look for at least the umbilical cord to fall off to ensure that it does not get submerged in water.

**The Where**

The biggest decision with giving the baby a bath is whereas the options would include a baby bath (if one was purchased), a regular bath, or the sink. Either will be perfectly adequate, it will all just depend on what works best for the family. For parents who have a small space, purchasing a baby bathtub may not be a feasible option, and there is nothing wrong with that.

In those instances, it is best to stick to the bathtub or sink. In some cases, a parent can also give the baby a shower, by showering right along with them. A bath can be given to the baby by itself in the big tub, using small amounts of water, or by taking a bath with the baby. A bath can be a scary experience for a baby in the beginning and taking a bath with a parent could be a soothing experience.

However, for the parents that decided they would feel more comfortable with a baby bathtub, there are different options to consider:

- Bathtubs that work as sink inserts. They are usually flexible and fit into most standard-sized sinks. Since they go into a sink, they are perfectly at the height for a standing adult and does not require leaning over.
- Standard tubs are standalone bathtubs made to fit children of various sizes and can be placed on the ground or a table or counter.
- Convertible tubs which are standalone tubs that have the ability to convert from newborn to toddler use.
- Hammock bathtubs are just that, regular standalone bathtubs that come with a mesh hammock for babies that are unable to support themselves.
- The inflatable tub is a space saver as it is blown up with air like an outdoor small pool.

- A fold-up tub is also a space saver like the inflatable tub. It is usually a hard tub, but it folds for easy storage. Most of these tubs can also be used from the newborn stage through toddlerhood.
- A bucket tub is a plastic bin that resembles more of a bucket than it does a bathtub, but it is designed to hold the baby in an upright position, much like a sink could.

There is no right answer when it comes to choosing the right tub and it is something that can be held off until the baby has arrived since a baby does not get a bath the moment that they are home. One can go as fancy or as simple as they feel like, or not purchase one at all.

When moving forward with actually making the purchase, if, at all possible, it's best to research the different types of tubs and how they work, even asking others for testimonials on their tubs. This may help in narrowing down which of the tubs mentioned above would meet the needs of the family and the baby specifically.

## The How

Once the desired area is chosen, the essentials for a bath are much the same as they are for a top and tail. The items that are most needed are a change of diaper, clothes, towel, soft rag to wash the baby with, and gentle baby soap. Again, it is best to ensure that the area the baby is bathed in is a warm one to prevent any colds.

Whether the baby is using its own bathtub, a regular bathtub, or the sink, there needs to be no more than around two inches of water. This will be enough water to ensure that the baby is kept warm throughout the experience, but not enough that they may become fully submerged on their own. Some simple tips can be provided for a good bathing experience:

- Gather all of your things in the area chosen for changing baby whether that is a changing table or bed. This way, once the baby is washed there will be no reason to waste time, preventing the baby from becoming cold.
- Ensure that the baby is kept warm throughout the experience by placing a small towel on top of the baby during the bath. Periodically, warm the towel in the bathwater and only take it off as you wash each area.
- It is best to use baby soap sparingly. This is to prevent the baby's skin from drying out or risking any type of skin outbreak should they be allergic.
- Always keep at least one hand on the baby in case the baby starts to slip. Never leave the baby unattended in the bath. If you find yourself needing to walk away, take the baby with you.
- After the baby is bathed, moisturize the baby's skin using either a special baby lotion or coconut oil.

Though a bath can seem daunting sometimes, there are only a few quick steps that need to be followed. All in all, as parents you just have to ensure that the baby is being bathed in a safe environment that is not too hot. A bath can be given as sparingly or as many times in a week as you would deem necessary.

**The Benefits**

Generally speaking, baby's like to take baths as long as it is a relaxing process, that is why some parents tend to incorporate that into the night time routine as the baby starts getting older. There are certain benefits to bathing the baby, whether it is something that parents decide to do daily or only two or three times a week. These benefits are more than just a clean baby at the end of the day.

- It helps with the parent-baby bond. Bath time can become a special time in the day between the baby and the parent. Both of you have to be focused on each other, the baby on the parent that is bathing it and the parent on the baby. There is time to have skin to skin contact, especially if you choose to have a bath or shower with your baby. When being bathed by mom, babies also like to feed if they are breastfed, facilitating that bond together.
- Bathing can become a learning experience for the baby. There are plenty of different toys available for bath time that can help with baby's development such as learning shapes or colors. Babies also learn to use their imaginations in the tub and learn to play with the water for later use in a pool scenario.
- Relaxes a baby that has become agitated. Throughout the day, a baby can become overstimulated learning different things and growing. A nice calm bath with a parent helps the baby calm down before they are put to bed for the

night. It's also a good way to introduce a baby massage to be given after the bath with the use of moisturizers.

- It helps the baby get ready for bed. There is a reason that parents start to introduce a bath, whether recommended daily or not, into a bedtime routine. The warmth of the water and the calmness of the situation helps babies get ready for sleep.

**The Challenges**

Like anything in life, even something as simple as bathing a baby can come with its own set of challenges. It's important to remember that a bath does not need to take place daily if this is something that has become a source of contention. Since each baby grows at their own rate, sometimes it is best to allow the baby to let you know when they are ready for something, such as taking baths more often.

Though most babies take to a bath right away, there are some babies that are not fond of bath time. If the baby gets very agitated at bath time, it is a good idea to check some things off the list to determine the cause.

- Check the temperature of the water. The baby may not be happy as the water is either too hot or too cold.
- The next time you bathe the baby, feed the baby first to ensure it just isn't hunger that is causing them distress.
- Try giving the baby a bath after a nap, or not too long after to rule out whether the baby has just been overtired and in no mood for bathing.
- The baby may just not feel safe in the water on their own or want the company. Taking a bath or shower with the baby is also an option to try and rule out baby discomfort.

Unfortunately, there are those babies that no matter the effort on the part of the parents, are just not fond of baths and may not be for a while yet. If that is the case, the best thing to do is to give fewer baths, since newborns don't require many to begin with and to try and give them as quickly as possible. Undress the baby right beside the tub or sink to minimize the bathing process and possible amount of time they feel cold. Though the baby may cry, there is no reason to become discouraged. As time progresses, and the baby grows, baths will become an event that the family will look forward to, filled with bubbles, toys, and fun.

**Product Guidelines**

When the baby is born it is protected by the vernix, a white substance that the baby forms in utero which protects the skin from outside elements. It works like a very well-made moisturizer. Well, after the baby's first birth, whether it's a cleaning given by the hospital or one at home, that vernix disappears. From there, the care of the baby's skin falls on the parents and the products they use.

One product is not equal to another as studies have shown us in the past. Recently, there has been a rise in products that are mostly natural due to people's fear of chemicals. The same type of care should be given to the choice made by parents regarding the products they use on their babies.

As a result of studies performed on various chemicals and baby products, it has been determined that there are quite a few chemicals that people have been using on their babies without giving them a second thought. Products that we used to believe are safe, may no longer be considered so.

- Talc: this is a powdered mineral that is commonly used in baby powder, a product that had been considered a staple in every home with a baby. Though talc works great as a drying substance, hence it's used on baby bottoms, it has been proven to be a lung irritant.
- Fragrance: many products on the shelves, whether for babies or adults, have an added fragrance which is supposed to kill off the smell of the chemicals that are used to make the products itself. The problem with the use of the term is that it encompasses any chemicals that the company uses, without disclosing the information in depth. However, most of these fragrances are based on coal or petroleum. Due to their design, they linger on the skin and are a common cause of respiratory, neurological, skin, or eye damage. In some cases, there has been evidence that the use of such fragrances can lead children to develop asthma. The biggest problem here is that they linger, and babies tend to put things in their

mouths, their own skin being number one on the list.

- Propylene Glycol: this chemical allows the product to be easily absorbed by the skin which pretty much means that this product will open the pores of the baby and allow things to sink in further. As an added perspective, propylene glycol is also a substance used in the windshield wiper fluid.
- 1,4 -dioxane and ethylated surfactants: studies performed by the Environmental Working Group showed that as many as 57% of baby products are made with this substance. This substance is actually a by-product when ethylene oxide is used to make other chemicals less harsh, but it in and of itself is a carcinogen.
- Mineral oil: this substance is a by-product that happens when petroleum is processed making it act like a plastic wrap around the skin. This type of chemical is usually found in baby oil and should be avoided at all costs. A better

alternative is something along the lines of olive or coconut oil.

- Parabens: these chemicals are linked to various issues such as reproductive toxicity, hormone disruption, and skin irritation. Unfortunately, this is a substance that is found almost everywhere, even if the product is marketed at babies.
- Triclosan: this pertains more or less to any product that is labeled as being antibacterial. This substance is considered a carcinogen and is harmful to the environment.

Due to the fact that studies have been performed and determined the above list of chemicals as the top ones to avoid, there are plenty of options out there that can be considered chemical-free. In some instances, it is even best to forgo buying a "beauty" product altogether as there are safer alternatives. As mentioned above, instead of using something like baby oil, coconut oil is a great alternative. This is something that can be purchased right off the shelf of a grocery store and will most likely not cost much more than a baby moisturizer.

Now that a thorough review of what should be avoided has been done, there are a couple of things to look for when purchasing baby bath products.

- Fewer ingredients: the smaller the list of ingredients on the back of the product, the better the product will be. Partially, this is because you will be able to make a much more informed decision. Unless someone is particularly knowledgeable about all of the ingredients, it is best to go with the shorter list of chemicals you understand more.
- Eco-friendly: make the choice be a product that is friendly to the environment as a whole and not just the one person. This is because anything that you used to wash with, whether it be yourself

or your baby, gets washed down the drain and goes back into the environment.

- Unscented products: as mentioned above, fragrances carry chemicals that are harmful not just to the person, but the environment as well. It is best to go for the products that advertise themselves as being fragrance-free.
- "All-purpose" products: this could be products that are advertised as a body wash and shampoo in one, which most of the baby products are. This helps keep down your own cost of product and saves the environment in various ways.

An alternative to trying to buy products that you feel comfortable with is making your own. Do-it-yourself products are at an all-time high since people trust it more. If you make the product yourself, you will obviously be aware of what you have used to make it. It can also become cost-efficient in the long run as most of the products you will buy to combine together you will purchase in bulk.

It only makes sense that with the studies that have been performed in the very recent past, people would shy away from as many chemicals as possible. This is especially true of parents who want to ensure that their babies are taken care of as best as possible.

**Bath accessories**

Babies come with all sorts of adorable accessories for every portion of their day and bathing is no different. There are many small and big accessories out there that can be purchased for bath time that may make it more enjoyable for both the parent and the baby.

- A hooded towel: though, of course, a towel is necessary to dry off and keep the baby warm, hooded towels are a bit of a novelty. They come in all sorts of patterns, whether they turn your baby in a lion or an elephant and are usually purchased just for sheer decoration.

- Bath toys: though a baby will not be able to pick up any toys yet, they can provide a good distraction and source of bonding time. Most of the first baby bath toys to be purchased are squeezable toys that squirt water. It is best to buy those that have a removable top to ensure that they can be properly cleaned and that mold will not form on the inside.
- Cups: these are specifically cups that help rinse the baby, especially the baby's head which not all babies are a fan of. It can be a regular looking cup with a cute pattern or more of a novelty such as in the shape of a whale that spits water. This is something that can be used on the baby as they grow making washing the head a better experience for all.
- A thermometer: though an elbow will do just as well at checking the temperature of the

water before you place the baby in it, there are thermometers designed specifically to show you the temperature of the water in many different shapes. For example, some come in the shape of ducks or turtles that will even advise if the temperature is getting too hot.

- Knee pads: this is more specific for parents, but there are knee pads, and in some instances, a combination of knee pads and elbow pads, to help you kneel beside the tub in comfort and give the baby a bath.
- No-slip mat: this is a rubber mat that suctions to the bottom of the tub to help the baby from slipping around. This is also something that could be used by the whole family.

In the very beginning, bath toys and accessories are just a novelty, they are not necessarily things that are needed in order to actually bathe the baby. Some things such as baby toys or the no-split mat are something that can continue being used down the road as the baby grows into a toddler making the investment something worthwhile.

**Takeaway**

Bath time can become a good source of a bonding experience between the baby and its parents or caregivers. There is one uniform way in which to give a baby a bath as it can be given in an actual tub, a baby bathtub, or the sink. There are also many different baby bathtubs out there to choose from should parents take that route.

What is important to remember is that though a bath can be a bonding experience, it does not have to happen often. It is best for the baby's skin if they are not bathed daily so as not to strip the baby's skin of its natural moisture. This means that when the baby is bathed it is important to moisture afterward. As mentioned, this can also be a good time to provide the baby with a small massage.

All in all, bathing a baby can become a great and wholesome experience, but some babies still don't like to bathe. That does not mean that the parents have done anything wrong, as there are no right or wrong answers here, but the baby may just need more time to grow into the idea. Slowly and steadily, it can be introduced and any fears on the part of the parent of the baby can be overcome.

# Chapter 5:
# Caring for Newborn Belly Button

**The Umbilical Cord**

An umbilical cord is what connects the baby to its mother inside of the womb. The cord runs from a hole in the baby's stomach and is connected to the placenta allowing it to carry vital nutrients from mother to the baby. On average, an umbilical cord is twenty inches long and is made up of one vein and two arteries.

The vein in the umbilical cord is what carries the oxygenated blood and nutrients from mom to the baby. On the other hand, the arteries return the deoxygenated blood and any waste products from the baby back to the placenta. At the end of the pregnancy, the cord will also supply the baby with antibodies made by the mother which will help protect the baby for up to three months after their birth.

After a baby is born, the cord will be clamped off about three or four inches away from the belly of the baby with a plastic clip. Next, the cord is clamped off close to the placenta and cut somewhere between the two clamps. The umbilical cord will then turn in to a stump that is roughly two to three inches in length. With a vaginal birth, the mother's partner is able to cut the cord should they request to do so, otherwise, it will be either the nurse, doctor, or midwife.

*Possible Medical Cord Issues*

Though the risk of umbilical cord issues, before or during the birth, taking place are very minor, in some instances as small as one percent, they should still be mentioned. These are conditions that can only be diagnosed by a doctor, in some instances with the use of ultrasound technology while the mother is still pregnant. In the end, however, none of these would impact the care that is given to the umbilical cord stump once the baby is at home and resting.

- Umbilical cord prolapse: this happens when the cord slips into the birth canal ahead of the baby and may become pinched. If your water were to break at home, it is best to head into the hospital, not just to ward off any possible bacteria, but to ensure that you are being monitored by doctors as the water first has to break before this is ever possible.
- Single umbilical artery: this is diagnosed when one of the arteries of the umbilical cord is missing. Unfortunately, there is no known reason why this happens, therefore, it is not something that can be prevented.
- Vasa Previa: this condition happens when one or more blood vessels from either the umbilical cord or the placenta cross the cervix.

- Nuchal cord: is when the cord wraps itself around the baby's neck which can be seen on an ultrasound. Most of the time, babies with a nuchal cord are born quite healthy.
- Umbilical cord knots: usually these knots form into the umbilical cord in the beginning of the pregnancy when the baby is able to move around more freely. Knots can be diagnosed by your doctor during routine ultrasounds of the baby during pregnancy. In most cases, if one is diagnosed, to ensure that the baby and the mother stay safe, a c-section will be performed.
- Umbilical cord cysts: these are sacks that are full of fluid within the umbilical cord. They are not that common as only less than one percent off pregnancies are diagnosed with this. Any cyst that is diagnosed already in the third trimester does not pose a danger to the baby.

## Caring for a newborn belly button

The stump of the belly button will fall off on its own within five to fifteen days from the birth of the baby. Once the stump has fallen off, the belly button will fully heal within seven to ten days. At first, the cord may appear to be yellow in color and as it dries it will turn to a greyish, or even purple, color. Those are all quite normal, as it will eventually shrivel and turn in to a black color before it falls off.

Though doctors used to recommend that the base of the stump is cleaned with rubbing alcohol, that has since changed. Nowadays, doctors advise parents to leave the stump alone, allowing it to dry and fall off on its own. If you find that the stump, or the area nearby appears too wet, you may dry it very gently with something like a Q-Tip and check that the baby is normally clothed in something breathable like cotton.

The one thing that parents have to remember is to keep the area dry, which means no fully submerged baths until the cord is gone and the area has healed. To ensure that it is healed properly, it is best not to pick at the stump even if appears to be hanging on by a thread. As soon as it is ready, it will fall off on its own, giving way for the belly button to hear naturally.

In the context of keeping the area dry, it is best to allow the stump to have air time as often as is possible. This means that any diaper that a baby is wearing is either cut specifically to allow the stump freedom or folding the diaper right below it. If it is feasible, it is also good to allow the baby to have some naked time. During the naked time, it is best to ensure that the baby will not go cold, therefore, any room that they are kept in should be kept warm and away from any drafts. This does not have to be a long length of time as it can be for just a couple of minutes during the day.

## Possible Belly Button Problems

Besides leaving the cord to its own ministrations, the parent should be on the lookout for a possible infection. There are a couple of signs that would help distinguish if the stump or belly button is infected and require medical attention:

- The base of the stump appears to be overly red or becomes swollen
- The cord continued to bleed
- There is yellow ooze or discharge from the belly button
- It holds a foul smell
- The baby seems to be reacting in pain if it is grazed or touched

Since any infection of the umbilical cord can give rise to what is called omphalitis. Omphalitis an infection of the umbilical cord and it is considered a life-threatening condition. As such, it should be treated immediately. It is best to call the pediatricians office to get the next steps on a possible appointment or immediate care instructions.

Another condition that affects the umbilical cord is what is called an umbilical granuloma. It is a small nodule that is usually pink or red in color which has a persistent yellow-green discharge. With a granuloma, there will be no swelling, redness, or fever to indicate that there is in fact anything wrong. If it is suspected that the baby has a granuloma, it is best to bring the baby to their pediatrician. In most cases, it is treated with silver nitrate which cauterizes the area. Since there are no nerve endings there, there is no need to worry as the baby will not feel any pain.

Lastly, the one question that parents find themselves asking quite often is whether there is a way to ensure that their baby has what is considered an "innie" instead of an "outie" belly button. Though in the past people have placed a coin over the belly button to help it go in, it is in fact proven that this will not help. Since the best thing for the belly button is to be left alone to heal, placing something like a coin is definitely not advisable, nor does it actually work.

There are times when a belly button that protrudes outward, or the "outie", can be a sign of a problem. Sometimes, the formation of the belly button in such a way is a sign of what is called an umbilical hernia. An umbilical hernia happens when the intestines and the surrounding fat are protruding through the muscles of the stomach and push out under the belly button. Though it takes a medical professional to diagnose a hernia, it is generally painless and will resolve on its own within at most a few years.

## What to do with the stump?

As the stump of the umbilical cord starts to dry and wither away, everyone takes a different approach to the process and what that means later. Some parents will be overjoyed at finally being able to give their newborn a proper bath, one they hope is filled with love and giggles. There are those parents, however, that hope to save it, as they may other things.

For those parents that decide to put the stump somewhere other than the immediate garbage can, there are options for its safekeeping that are both practical and adorable.

- Scrapbook or memory book: this is the easiest approach as there are many options out there that have space for the umbilical stump to be placed. Before taping it in, however, be sure that it is thoroughly dried or place it in a baggie if you are not sure.

- Bury it: some cultures have adapted the burying of the stump from generation to generation. There are also moms that have started the practice even if it is not their cultural norm by burying the stump somewhere and placing a plant on top whether a tree, bush, or flowers.
- Jewelry: much as breastmilk can be turned in to jewelry, so can the umbilical stump. There are companies out there that will transform the stump into a beautiful looking piece of jewelry that can be worn by the mother. Jewelers that specialize in this type of work can make various pieces out of the stump such as a necklace or ring.
- Frame it: this option could include more than just the umbilical stump. A shadowbox is a great idea for placing baby items into and hanging it on a wall for either personal or public display.
- Toy (or something of the like): this means sewing the stump into a favorite toy or lovey, most likely once the child outgrows the toy. This allows

the parents to keep the toy and give it to their child once they are grown.

All of these options are safe and are something that can be passed down to the child once the time is right as they won't understand the significance until they are much older.

The option to save the stump is not for everyone, of course, and no one should feel that they need to do so. Though it may be an amazing thing to look back on in later years, it may be more amazing for the mother rather than anyone else like the grown child.

**Takeaway**

When mom and baby are still one, with the baby safely tucked away inside the womb, the umbilical cord is what gives the baby life. Though there are some medical issues that can happen with this life-giving cord, they are very few and far between and do not need any further thought unless brought up by the doctor.

The important thing to remember about the stump and the belly button is that for the most part, it takes care of itself, as long as it receives some gentle treatment. It has been designed to fall off on its own within a couple of days from the birth of the baby as long as it is kept dry and not overly restricted. If anything at all looks amiss, it is best to contact the pediatrician right away for further information on treatment.

# Chapter 6: Clothing baby

Clothing a baby, whether they are for a boy or a girl, is one of the tasks that parents look forward to the most. The outfits that are available for any gender are absolutely adorable, however, there are so many choices and so many things to keep in mind when making purchases.

When it comes to newborns, preparation really does matter, hence the institution of having a baby shower. Not only is a time for others to come and join the parents on such a joyous occasion and show their support, but it is also a wonderful way for parents to prepare as much as possible for their bundle of joy that will join them in the world soon.

Clothing is one of the most purchased items for a baby shower whether the parents have found out the gender ahead of time, or they are remaining gender-neutral until the baby is born. What this means for the parents is that because it is difficult to predict the sizes that will be needed once the baby is born, it is best to buy the minimum at first as others will have already added on to the pile of newborn clothes whether we asked them to or not.

## Types of outfits available and how many needed

Before either shopping for the clothes ourselves or placing them on to a baby shower registration, be cognizant of the sizes that are out there. First and foremost, each brand has specifics when it comes to the sizes of their clothes, therefore, it is best to look closely. Most brands will actually list not just the size on the tag, but how big baby has to be in order to fit into those sizes best. There is usually a weight and length measurement provided on the tag underneath the size pointing you in the right direction.

In the first few weeks of life, newborns will grow exponentially. At first, the baby is growing in order to make up the weight that they lost after birth, and then later they will continue to grow, moving up from one size to another pretty quickly. By around five months or so, the baby should have doubled in weight, definitely outgrowing most of their first baby clothes by that time.

Remember, some babies are born on the smaller side which means that they will fit into preemie clothes, and some are born a little later which means that they will outgrow the newborn size relatively fast. Therefore, the number of clothes that you will need to settle on depends on the number of times in a week that you will want to focus on doing laundry. Based on the recommendations below, if you plan on doing laundry only once in a week, it is best to double the amount recommended. If you wash clothes every day, as is in some families, you can take the amount recommended and cut it by half.

- Bodysuits or Rompers: these types of outfits are usually the staple in any baby closet. During the summer months, they can be used as a quick light outfit, and in the winter, they can be used as a base to keep the baby warm since they do come in a long-sleeve option. The recommended amount to have on hand is about seven.
- 
- Pants: at the newborn age, most babies do not wear pants unless it is chilly outside, therefore it is good to have at least three pairs on hand.
- Hats: there are plenty of hats that come with outfits and do not have to be purchased separately, however, since newborns are still learning to regulate their body temperature, it is best to have two on hand for the first weeks.

- Socks: since babies cannot walk, they don't really need socks unless it is winter and exceptionally cold. It is best to have around five pairs of socks and it is best to get them all in one color. With as small as baby socks are, they tend to get lost pretty quickly as well.
- Swaddles: though these are not necessarily considered clothing that baby will wear out, it is best to have two or three on hand if you are choosing to swaddle the baby in the middle of the night. Do your research on different types of swaddles out there, however, since they can be very specific to be baby size, meaning that if the baby is born on the smaller end, they will most likely need to wait to use it.
- Sleepers (pajamas): these come in footed, non-footed, or gowns options and it is best to have around four on hand of any of these. These are great for playtime or can be used inside a swaddle as well. They are cozy and great insulators for the baby during colder days or nights.

- Sweaters: this includes any sweatshirt type shirts. It is best to have two sweaters on hand whether they are cardigan or zippered. Since the baby cannot be placed into a car seat with a jacket or bunting, this can be used as an added layer to ward off the cold.
- Mittens: depending on how much the baby leaves the house during the colder months, it is best to have two pairs of warmer mittens on hand. For year-round use, there are mittens out there specifically designed so that the baby doesn't cut themselves with their fingernails until they can be cut. It is best to have two of those on hand as well.

Specifically, for the winter months, it is best to have the following on hand as well:

- Winter coat: this can be either an actual jacket or a bunting which may be easier to use for a newborn. Only one of these is needed, but be aware that in most of these outfits the baby should not be placed into a car seat. Due to the bulkiness of such clothing, the car seat straps will not sit close enough to the chest and could cause the baby to fly out of the seat in case of an accident. They do come in handy when taking the baby for a walk in a stroller, however.

- Slippers (booties): these will not be used for walking, but a pair can come in handy if it is cold and baby's feet need to be kept warm outside, such as if the baby is not using a bunting but a jacket instead.

- 
- Other options:
- Fancy clothing: this is usually purchased on an as-needed basis since situations such as these cannot always be prepared for ahead of time. For a girl, this will usually include something like a dress, a bow, and stockings. For a boy, this would include a suit, shirt, and tie or bow tie.

- Baby bows: this more specific to baby girls and is used mostly for decorative purposes. They come in all sorts of sizes, from small to bows that are larger than the baby's head. Each of them has something special about it. This is not necessarily a practical piece of clothing, but for baby girls, it can be very adorable.

*Swimming:*

Swimming is a fun past time for both adults and children, and even babies. Though of course, they won't be able to swim just yet, there is nothing that says babies cannot be brought either to a pool or the beach. As is, a baby will need some type of swimsuit to wear, and with so many options it can be overwhelming.

- Rashguard: can be purchased for both boys and girls. This can be either a shirt or a one-piece that resembles a romper. They are made of a specialized material to be used in the sun.
- Swim trunks: are miniature versions of swim trunks that you can buy for an adult. The

material is usually made with UPF 50 for sun protection. Most of the time, they will also have a mesh on the inside, however, a baby will still need a diaper (preferably one made for swimming, so it is not as ultra-absorbent as regular diapers).

- One-piece swimsuits: are a great comfortable design for girls, giving them freedom and comfort at the same time.
- Two-piece bikinis: though this is also an option for girls, they may not be the best for a newborn. The reason for this is that babies need to be covered more to be protected from the sun and other elements around them. Purchasing a one-piece instead will keep your baby girl warm and protected at the same time.

Another tip for the sun, whether boy or girl, is to use a sun hat. This will ensure that the baby's face and neck are protected from the sun before they reach an age where they can use suntan lotion. Hats designed for the pool or the beach are also made of a material that is around UPF 50 to ensure that the baby does not get too much sun.

*Small tips:*

When purchasing any of the baby clothes mentioned above, it is best to keep some things in mind to make the baby as comfortable as possible. Remember, a baby spends most of their time asleep or just laying down and it is best to purchase clothing that will make them comfortable.

- Purchase clothing that is seasonally appropriate such as short sleeves onesies in the summer and long-sleeves in the winter.
- Buy clothing that is comfortable such as no large buttons.
- Avoid clothing with a hood or a collar. This is partly because a hood can get stuck or wrapped around the baby, and the other is due to the fact

that both pieces of clothing would touch the baby's cheek. In the beginning, when the baby's cheek is touched it triggers the rooting reflex which would make the baby constantly search for food.

- Unless the opening is big enough, avoid buying things that have to go over the head. This is mostly for your own comfort as parents rather than for the babies. That is to say, keep in mind that anything that is tight going over the head will be tight being taken off which means if the baby has a poop blow-out, you might smear the baby in it unless you want to cut off the piece of clothing. As an added tip, some onesies come with shoulder flaps which extend the neckline and allow the onesie to be taken off through the bottom as opposed to the top.
- It is best to stick to clothing that is soft, easy to clasp (such as buttons on a onesie that are between the legs) with built-in feet. This will minimize the amount of work that has to be done

every time that a baby has to have a diaper change and the number of lost socks.

## Clothing the baby at the hospital

Depending on how the baby is born, whether vaginal or c-section, will determine the next steps, however, in the end, the baby is always placed into a newborn shirt and a swaddle, with a small hat on for warmth. Though parents are allowed to bring their own outfits, and some choose to, there is actually no need.

Part of the reason that is best to leave the baby in the clothes provided by the hospital is the ease of access. Throughout the day, each day before discharge, nurses will be checking in on the baby to make sure that the baby is doing well. There will also be a pediatrician stopping by at least once a day. By leaving the baby in the hospital shirt and the swaddle blanket, nurses are able to come in and do their job quickly and efficiently without disturbing the baby too much.

If you choose to bring outfits for the baby to the hospital to wear before going home, it is best to keep it simple, such as footed sleepers or onesies. It is best to bring a few just in case there are any diaper accidents. Since the baby will still be swaddled to help them sleep through the newborn startle reflex, they do not have to be overly warm outfits so that the baby does not overheat.

One more thing that the hospital provides is the standard-issue blankets that are white, pink, and blue and have become known almost everywhere. Though parents have been told not to take those home, plenty of them do for sentimental reasons. With the hospitals providing these blankets for generations, they have become a staple of the newborn wardrobe and baby's first pictures. They are also specifically designed to be just the right size and shape to be a swaddle for the baby.

## Coming home outfit

Choosing a coming home outfit has become a rather lengthy and involved process, with parents striving to choose the outfit they believe is best. The choice of what to bring the baby home in is completely up to the parents, though some strive to make the outfit more memorable than the rest.

With many companies out there targeting this type of market, there are plenty of choices from practical to adorable. Some parents have even personalized the outfit with the chosen name of the baby, or a small saying or poem.

There is no right or wrong answer, however, what should be kept in mind is that you will never know the exact size that the baby will be born. Unless you plan on purchasing different outfits (or even the same one) in different sizes, it is also good to have a backup in case the baby is either bigger or smaller than was expected.

Even if adorable is what you are going for, remember to keep the baby comfortable as well. Comfort is going to be key for the baby and parents on one of those most important days. Going home is already a new experience for the baby, and can be quite overwhelming, therefore, it is best to make the transition from hospital to home as easy as possible. Also, once the baby is home, most of the time they will end up going back to sleep, so choosing something more comfortable will minimize the amount of fuss needed once there.

To top it off, remember, that this type of outfit will only be worn by the baby most likely once, if not just a small handful of times. Since outfits like these can be pricier than the rest, if money is a factor, it may be best to go with something more practical, which of course can still be flattering and memorable for the occasion.

**Tips for dressing a newborn**

Dressing a baby for the first time can be an intimidating undertaking, but it can be overcome. Since a newborn is not the wiggle worm that it will once become, the process of dressing a newborn is much easier with some practice. There are a few short tips that can be considered in order to make the process easy in the hospital and at home.

- Dress the baby on a changing table or a wider surface such as a bed or the floor. Once the baby is able to start rolling over, which won't be for a couple of months, it is best to avoid places such as a bed to prevent the baby from taking a tumble, therefore, it might be best to get in the habit of doing it somewhere else right away.

- In the beginning, babies will not be able to pull away from things that cover their faces, so it is best to dress them in clothes that fit the baby and do not wrap around their neck too tight. Make sure that anything decorative such as buttons is secured tightly and won't fall off as the baby is wearing their outfit.
- Due to the wiggly nature of babies, it is best to reach through either the sleeves or the legs before pulling the limb through. This will minimize the chance that the baby may get stuck or hurt.
- Make it a bonding moment. This can be done by talking or singing with the baby. In some instances, it may make the process of getting dressed easier once the baby is bigger and starts to have opinions of their own.

Dressing a baby does not have to be as heart-stopping as it might sound. Babies are a lot tougher than most people think that they are, and with some practice, it is possible to get the hang of it. Parents can become experts in no time and will gladly branch out their baby's wardrobe as time goes on.

## Choosing type of diaper; disposable or cloth

The decision whether to use cloth or disposable diapers is another big decision in the life of a parent and, as with many other choices, there is no right or wrong answer. The decision will vary from family to family based on a number of different circumstances which may make one easier to use than the other.

There are no real differences between cloth and disposable diapers except for someone's preference. It is perfectly acceptable to also make that decision once the baby has been born and it is easier to see what the routine will look like and whether it will fit the family. It may also be a better option to wait until the baby's arrival as not all cloth diapers are made equal. Disposable diapers will come in all sorts of sizes and if you find that you have the wrong one, you can either purchase more or exchange what you have. Cloth diapers, on the other hand, start at a certain rage of weight the baby must meet, meaning that they may not work for each baby right away.

One of the biggest decision-making differences between the two is the total cost. The average cost of diapering one child can run up to $3,000 for around two years. The price goes up, of course, if it is taking the baby a little longer to potty train than the moment, they hit two years. However, cloth diapering can run around $1,000 total if you plan on doing laundry yourself. If you plan on outsourcing diaper laundry, the total price will end up running similar to those of disposable diapers.

It is important to remember though, that the total price of the diapers when using cloth has to be paid upfront. This is due to the fact that a newborn will most likely end up being changed around ten times a day. In order to be able to keep up with the demand, you will have to purchase enough diapers to last those ten times for at least two days so that you are not forced to do laundry more than once a day. Of course, if you do not want to, or have the ability to, do laundry once a day, you will end up needing more diapers. This could equate to around twenty to thirty cloth diapers on hand.

If you plan on moving forward with disposable diapers, that cost can be spread out over time allowing you to save for those week by week, but of course, as mentioned earlier, the total cost of the diapering will end up running about twice as much.

The biggest benefit of cloth diapers is that you are able to use them on any subsequent sibling. With the proper care and cleaning, they can last for years and be used for multiple siblings once one is potty trained. In some instances, if parents have decided they are done having children, it is possible to resell them to another set of parents. There are plenty of different platforms that parents frequent, such as Facebook Marketplace, that make it easier to sell such items that are still in good condition.

Since most cloth diapers have a minimum weight recommendation before they fit the baby properly, this is something that can be held off until the baby is born. This will allow you time to decide which ones will work best for you and your family as well as which ones will fit the baby how quickly. If in the meantime you decide that disposable diapering will work better, you have not spent the money on cloth diapering before you were sure of which avenue to take.

Convenience is also something that is a factor when choosing which is the best for your family. Disposable diapers can be move convenient, especially when on the go, therefore, it is good to keep in mind that cloth diapering can be something done strictly at home. However, there are parents who find cloth diapering a little cumbersome. Though cloth diapers have come leaps and bounds from what they used to be back in the day, there are still quite a bit of pieces that need to be juggled in order to make it work.

Disposable diapers are a one and done deal, meaning that they can be thrown out the moment that they've been soiled, straight into the garbage with the entire mess. Sometimes, even the outfit goes with if it was a big enough explosion. That is not the case, however, with cloth diapers. They require washing, but in the meantime, they have to be stored in a bag, or laundry hamper, that is specifically designed to hold those diapers as they are wet and most likely soiled.

A baby can pee up to twenty times a day, and within those twenty breastfed babies will poop at least three times a day and formula-fed babies around one to four times. What this means for the parent, is the need to store all of those diapers in between washes. If parents are on the go, storing and bringing those back home can become quite cumbersome, and some might find it quite gross.

Some have also made the claim that cloth diapers are better for the environment, swaying parents to go down that route. However, that is not as clear cut as it seems. Yes, disposable diapers do fill up landfills and do not always degrade the way that we would like them to, however, cloth diapers require a lot of cleaning which of course requires energy and water.

If it is hard to commit to the purchase of cloth diapers upfront, as you need to make a big enough purchase for the whole thing to make sense, and you do not personally have anyone to ask advice of, there are online and community groups that either provide that much needed advice or testimonials, but also rentals. There are boutiques out there that give the ability to rent diapers in different brands to see which ones would work best when considering cloth diapering. This helps with making the ultimate decision to spend or not spend the money.

The decision on what would work best for the family lies only with the parents, however, there is no right or wrong answer. If you find that cloth diapering is not for you, there is no reason to feel as if there has been a wrong decision made, even though some would make you feel otherwise.

## Takeaway

Overall, there are many options out there when it comes to clothing the baby, from what to bring to a hospital, their coming home outfit, how many clothes they should have in the beginning, to whether to include cloth diapers or disposable diapers in the whole ensemble.

Though there are certain guidelines that can be provided, such as the recommended amount of articles of clothing, there are no right or wrong answers when it comes to what the parents decide. Most of the time, it will be trial and error that parents have to learn to cope with. You can purchase or be gifted as many little outfits as you choose, whether your baby ends up wearing them all or not.

You can go either practical or pretty no matter what gender your baby is, and that is quite alright. Many parents, especially mothers, love to dress their child up in special outfits and that is their choice. A baby is a newborn only once in their life and you can make that time special for you, whatever that means.

# Chapter 7:
# Caring for a Circumcision

Circumcision is a very personal decision that should not be influenced by anyone, but it has become a highly volatile topic among parents. It is, of course, a decision that can in no way be reversed, but should be discussed before the birth of the baby, even if the gender is not known right away.

Though statistics vary by region, in the United States around 55% to 65% of all newborn baby boys undergo circumcision. This is a procedure that is common mostly in North America, Africa, and the Middle East. It is not a common procedure performed in South America, Asia, or Europe.

If the baby is being born in the hospital, the decision on whether to circumcise or not should be made known to the hospital nurse. As it is the ob-gyn that will perform the procedure most likely within a day or two of the birth, they will be made aware immediately.

If the baby is not being born in the hospital, contact your pediatrician for further guidance on how to set up the procedure. It is best, however, not to wait too long if you would like to have your boy circumcised since the longer you wait, the more painful it is.

**First, what is it and why?**

*What is it?*

Anatomically, boys are born with a layer of skin called the foreskin covering the head of the penis that is called the glans. Circumcision is the surgical removal of the foreskin of the penis. This is the layer of skin that covers the head of the penis. It is a straight forward procedure that is performed by the obstetric gynecologist that delivered the baby if the delivery was in the hospital.

Usually, this procedure is performed within the first ten days of the baby's life to minimize any risks and pain, though usually if the baby is born in hospital doctors try to do it within a day or two.

The choice to have a son circumcised can vary greatly, but some of the most common reasons are:

• Health benefit: specifically, the prevention of urinary tract infections (UTI) as well as the decreased possibility of contracting sexually transmitted diseases (STD). For uncircumcised males, there are bacteria that get caught underneath the skin which can lead to UTI. It is believed that with the removal of that skin, there is a fewer risk of having a UTI. There has also been research performed which came to the conclusion that males that have been circumcised have a smaller chance of contracting HIV from an infected partner, however, as with most things, more research is still needed.

- Appearance: if, for instance, the father of the child has been circumcised, parents might be more inclined to do the same in order to make sure that they do not look different.
- Religion or culture: in some cultures, or religions, circumcision is something that has been a part of the practice for many centuries, for example, in the Muslim or Jewish communities.

*Why not?*

Some parents choose not to move forward with circumcision, due to:

- Pain: parents decide not to have this procedure done to spare the baby any pain as this is something that will have to heal over some time. Though the baby is given an anesthetic before the procedure itself takes place, it is still a wound that has to heal when the baby is taken home.

- Risk: as with any other surgical procedure, there is also a risk when circumcising a child. Though they are very rare, complications are something that can happen and will include either bleeding, infection or scarring. To mitigate these types of problems, it is best to ensure that it is a medical professional who is well trained in this procedure that will carry out the circumcision.
- Autonomy: some parents believe that this is a decision that should be made by the child once they are old enough to make it, however, this is something that is quite painful to do once the child is older, especially as they are nearing adulthood. At that time, there is also a bigger possibility of complications arising.

*Methods*

To assist you in the decision on whether to have your boy circumcised, it is best to familiarize yourself with the different methods that the procedure is performed. These methods are through the use of the Gomco circumcision clamp, the Mogen circumcision clamp, or the PlastiBell circumcision device. In the U.S. however, the Gomco clamp is one of the most commonly used devices, but you can always check that with the doctor that will be performing the procedure.

- Of the three types of devices, the Gomco clamp is one of the most difficult to use even if it provides better cosmetic results. It is the hardest because the partially cut foreskin must be threaded between the bell and the clamp before the actual clamp is tightened to make the cut. This also comes with some bleeding.
- The Mogen clamp is the next most commonly used and mostly within the Jewish community. This device is the one that is

generally regarded as the quickest and the one that produces the least discomfort.

- The PlastiBell is very easy in its use, but it must remain on the penis until the foreskin becomes necrotic and it falls off. This process may take seven to ten days which means that many parents tend to dislike this type of device.

Electrocautery is the one type of method that is not recommended which is something commonly used by urologists. This is not a recommended method due to the studies that have been performed which revealed that there are possible complications such as the transected penile head (or cut), severe burns, or meatal stenosis (a narrowing of the urethral opening, or the hole at the top).

Knowing what the procedure looks like beforehand may ease the decision-making process one way or another. Some parents are afraid to make the decision because they never know what they are getting in to, but that should have eased the picture that the mind creates when it comes to circumcision.

*The Checklist*

Before a circumcision is performed there are a couple of things that have to be checked off the proverbial checklist to ensure that it is safe to have it performed. Usually, these things are done by the doctor, but as parents, it is also good to keep on top of the process from start to finish.

- The baby must be examined by a pediatrician or another doctor who can provide the same level of care to determine that all is well.
- The baby must be full-term (or close to) how is healthy and has been stable.
- The penis itself must be of normal size without any defects.
- It must be determined by the doctor that if the procedure is carried out, the skin of the shaft

does not move forward to cover the head of the penis due to excess abdominal fat.

- Determine that there is no risk of a bleeding disorder that may prove counterproductive to the correct healing of the circumcision.

- A vitamin K shot must have been administered to the baby upon birth to help with clotting.

**The How**

The circumcision procedure lasts usually no more than ten minutes and is done within ten days of the baby's birth in the nursery. The quick procedure will see that your son is lying on his back with arms and legs restrained to prevent undue movement. The doctor will inject an anesthetic into the base of the penis after the area has been fully cleansed. Sometimes the anesthetic is actually provided in the form of a cream.

Once the foreskin is removed with whichever method your doctor has deemed best, the penis will be covered with a topic antibiotic or some petroleum jelly and wrapped in gauze.

For boys or adults that are older, the procedure looks much the same, however, it might be performed under general anesthesia and it might take longer to heal. There are also greater risks of different complications taking place in older males, hence why the push for it to be done when the baby is born.

**Caring for the circumcision**

Due to the fact that circumcision is a surgical procedure, it will require a certain level of care once it is performed. This is to ensure that the risk of contracting any infections is minimized and that it heals without needing any medical intervention. Normally, the staff at the hospital where it is done will go through the process with you, however, here are things to keep in mind.

- During each diaper change, without touching it as much as is possible, inspect the penis to see that it does not appear infected.
- No thorough cleaning will need to be performed so as not to cause any undue pain.
- Before replacing the diaper, apply a liberal amount of petroleum jelly either straight on to the penis or on to a gauze that you will place over the penis inside the diaper. This is to ensure that the wound does not dry out or get stuck to the fabric of the diaper.
- If any stool does get on to the penis, since as a newborn stool can be very loose, use a soft cotton towel and nothing more than soap and water to clean off the dirty area.

- Usually, circumcision will be healed fully within about seven to ten days. In the meantime, you will find that the head of the penis will appear red and there will be what looks like a yellow fluid. Both of these are quite normal as the penis heals from the procedure.
- If during your inspection you find that the penis is not healing within the specified amount of time, has turned a different color, or has crusted over, it is best to contact the pediatrician office immediately for further instructions.

Once the penis has healed from the procedure, cleaning it on a daily basis will require nothing more than soap and water during bath time. If during a diaper change, you find that the stool has made its way up, a wet wipe will suffice.

If you find that there is some skin left over, do not attempt to pull the skin back on your own as this could cause more harm than good. Most of the time this skin will detach on its own as it does for a boy who has been left uncircumcised. If there are any questions on the way that it healed, or if it looks correct, ask the pediatrician.

**What if I don't do it?**

If you choose to not circumcise your son, let your wishes be known at the hospital while you are being admitted for delivery. It is best to ensure that all medical staff is aware of your request, however, no one should move forward with any procedures as you would have to sign your approval.
The care for an uncircumcised penis is a little different overall, however, it is not any more difficult than if the procedure was done.

- When dirty, such as during a runny stool, wash the penis with soap and water, nothing else is required.
- Do not under any circumstances, pull back on the foreskin. This used to be advised to new parents, however, it was found to be doing more

harm to boys than it was beneficial. It's important to remember that most likely the skin will not fully pull back until the boy is older.

- As your boy ages, remember to teach him the importance of washing the area with soap and water as by that point in time he should be able to gently start moving the foreskin back to clean properly.

There is nothing wrong with leaving a boy uncircumcised. Studies have shown that more parents are starting to shy away from the practice for various reasons. The care for a penis that has not been circumcised is not any more difficult as mentioned below as there are only key pieces to remember.

**Takeaway**

Circumcision is a personal choice on the part of the parents and as with everything else, there is technically no right answer. Above are some of the key points on what circumcision is and what it looks like as well as the criteria the baby boy needs to meet before having it performed.

Since it is a surgery, it is best to discuss all the information that you have learned with the doctor who will be performing the surgery such as the ob-gyn or the pediatrician. If you choose to move forward, the medical staff at the hospital will teach you how to care for the wound once you go home, but it does not take long to heal at all. Within ten days or so, everything has healed and will no longer require any special care.

If you choose to uncircumcised, there are no other steps that need to be done besides educating yourself on how to care for it during bath time or diaper changes. Nowadays, it is best to leave the skin as is, as it will finally retract on its own as the boy grows and that is the most important thing to remember. Again, this is something that can be asked the hospital staff before going home with the baby for the first time.

# Conclusion

Thank you for making it through to the end of *Newborn Care Basics: Baby Care Tips For New Moms*, let's hope it was informative and able to provide you with all of the tools you need to achieve your goals whatever they may be. As with many topics, there is a wealth of information out there to learn, with this book being just the beginning.

The next step is to further your knowledge on any of the topics listed above such as discussing important information with your chosen pediatrician or ob-gyn. There are other books available online or at your local library, as well as community groups that could point you in the right direction. Don't be afraid to reach out and generate more information that you could use later.

The most important thing to remember when caring for a newborn is that not everything is a one size fits all. Not every baby is the same just as not every parent is the same, and there is nothing wrong with that. Based on the knowledge that you have gained after reading this book, choose the options that best suit the needs of your baby and your family. Be it, the type of clothes you choose, whether you move forward with cloth or disposable diapers, or bathe your baby daily. As a parent, you will no doubt do your best and continue to learn things along the way that will help you bond with your baby and watch them continue to grow beyond the newborn stage.

**Do let us know how this book helped you by leaving a review. This will encourage eager parents to make the right purchase. Happy Parenting!**

# *Other Books by Lisa Marshall*

## Easy Newborn Care Tips

*Proven Parenting Tips For Your Newborn's Development, Sleep Solution And Complete Feeding Guide*

## Newborn Care Basics

*Baby Care Tips For New Moms*

## Toddler Discipline Tips

*The Complete Parenting Guide With Proven Strategies To Understand And Managing Toddler's Behavior, Dealing With Tantrums, And Reach an Effective Communication Communication With Kids*

# **Becoming a Dad**

## ***The First-Time Dad's Guide to Pregnancy Preparation***
## ***(101 Tips For Expectant Dad)***

# **Positive Parenting Solutions 2-in-1 Box Set**

### ***Easy Newborn Care Tips + Toddler Discipline Tips***

### ***The OffIcial Parenting Guide To Raising Your Spirited Child***

# *Follow Lisa Marshall*

**\* Subscribe to Our Newsletter and Get <u>FREE</u> resources!**
<u>SUBSCRIBE HERE</u>
**copy** <u>http://bit.ly/becomingadad</u> **paste**

**Download one audiobook for FREE!**
You can download the audiobook version of all my books for FREE just by signing up for a FREE 30-days Audible trial! Just click on the following direct link and then find the audiobook you wish to listen...
<u>AUDIOBOOK US</u>   or   <u>AUDIOBOOK UK</u>

**Follow us on Facebook**
<u>https://www.facebook.com/LisaMarshallAuthor</u>

**Note:** If you have purchased the paperback format then you need to write this link on your browser search bar.

**Finally, if you found this book useful in any way, a review on Amazon is always appreciated!**

465

www.ingramcontent.com/pod-product-compliance
Lightning Source LLC
Chambersburg PA
CBHW020238030426
42336CB00010B/522